M000050048

Psychiatry at Harborview:

Community • Compassion • Care

SHARON ROMM, MD

Clinical Associate Professor
Department of Psychiatry and Behavioral Sciences
University of Washington
Seattle, WA

LIGER
PRESS

LIGER PRESS

Copyright © 2021 by Sharon Romm, MD
All rights reserved

ISBN: 978-1-09834-658-4 (paperback)
978-1-09834-659-1 (eBook)

With appreciation for

Jürgen Unützer, MD, MPH, MA
Professor and Chair, Department of Psychiatry and Behavioral Sciences
University of Washington

and

Mark Snowden, MD, MPH
Chief of Psychiatry, Harborview Medical Center
Professor, Department of Psychiatry and Behavioral Sciences
Vice Chair of Clinical Affairs
University of Washington

and

All my colleagues at Harborview

and

Remembering Oliver Black
(1957 – 2019)

Although many colleagues were interviewed, the author spoke directly with no patient. All patient vignettes are either modeled on a single or composite of actual persons. If a patient is described, their identifying information has been sufficiently altered so an individual cannot be recognized.

Table of Contents

Foreword

Dr. Sharon Romm has worked in the Psychiatric Intensive Care Unit at Harborview Medical Center for more than XX years. In this role, she has been at the forefront of our mission to develop unique and innovative programs for patients with complex psychiatric and medical illnesses.

When I joined Harborview in 2014 as its executive leader, I was drawn by its comprehensive mission to serve vulnerable communities and its pioneering work in many fields. What strikes me most about Dr. Romm and her colleagues is their ability to see beyond disease labels, such as anxiety disorders, schizophrenia, suicidality and self-destructive behaviors. Instead, they treat every individual as a person who is deserving of care and dignity.

Let me illustrate this point with a story that Dr. Romm published in the American Journal of Psychiatry. In this touching vignette, she described the transformation of an angry, psychotic substance abuser to a gentle, kindly man facing his last days. But this transformation extended beyond the patient to his care team. In her last conversation with him, she said, "You have given us the privilege and the joy of caring for you."

As both an academic medical center managed by UW Medicine and a county-owned safety-net hospital, Harborview has a rich history of growth and innovation. In Psychiatry at Harborview, you will discover the depth of services that we provide to people with mental illnesses. You will also come to know the expert teams that surround each individual with care, compassion and community.

Dr. Romm brings to this history her gifts as a storyteller. Once you conclude this chronicle, you will be amazed and gratified, as I am continually, to know that Psychiatry at Harborview is an incredible asset for our community and those it serves.

Paul Hayes, RN
Chief Executive Officer Harborview Medical Center
October 2020

Author's Note

Psychiatry at Harborview presents an exceptional service at a special hospital. Harborview, home to one quarter of the 1,000 employees of the University of Washington's Department of Psychiatry and Behavioral Sciences, provides unparalleled care to all.

Harborview is the most unique hospital of its kind in the Northwest and, possibly, farther afield as well. Its excellent reputation is reinforced every day. Harborview serves patients from all walks of life: from those blessed with good income, career, and clean clothing to those who have no home let alone a reliable place to sleep, a change of undergarments, or a guaranteed meal. Harborview sees no differences and has no favorites. It doesn't matter if a patient is unwashed or undocumented or underfed. All who are in need of care get the very best.

I came to Harborview as an adventure, planning to stay a year, and remained for two decades. I didn't choose Seattle for the mountains or weather; Seattle simply wasn't my East Coast home. What kept me here was this extraordinary hospital with its sense of community spirit, its commitment to quality, and knowing that everyone is on the same team with the same mission.

Harborview arose from a two-story wooden building with six beds in an out-of-town marshland setting and has grown to a sizable institution with 5,000 employees. This large facility now commands the respect of the general public and the medical establishment.

My psychiatry department is special. It represents every imaginable aspect of our field, offering an impressive array of services. We are proud to present specialists in treating the acutely ill; specialists who attend to a large number of outpatients; specialists in chemical dependency and psychotherapy; and we have talented researchers, psychologists, pharmacists and social workers who contribute their skills. Also on our team are extraordinary nurses who, like their provider colleagues, are always ready to go above and beyond the call. Work extra hours, see extra patients? Everyone pitches in when the need arises.

If you're a psychiatrist, perhaps this book will inspire you to join us and become part of an energetic and progressive team. No matter what your interests in the field, there may be a place for you. Read this book and see what Harborview psychiatry can offer. Read patients' and providers' stories of success and occasional disappointment and you'll learn about a real and humane institution.

If you're not a psychiatrist, you will still find it a treat to take a journey through our department. You'll meet an impressive selection of people who will inspire you with their accomplishments, enthusiasm, and excellence.

Welcome—and enjoy your visit with us!

1

Beginnings: Harborview's Story

After separating from Oregon in 1853 and before achieving statehood in 1889, Washington became an independent territory. An early ruling made its counties responsible for all "poor, sick and homeless people whose relatives could not support them." As a result, in 1877, King County opened its "Poor Farm" in the marshlands along the banks of the Duwamish River south of Seattle.

Within the two-story wooden structure of the Poor Farm, six beds were designated "King County Hospital" and staffed, at first, by three French Canadian Sisters of Providence nurses transported by paddleboat from Portland to Seattle. The hospital later moved to downtown Seattle and was renamed Providence Hospital. Due to friction between its management and the county commissioners, the facility had to return to the old Poor Farm site. By 1894, however, a new 125-bed King County Hospital was opened in Seattle's Georgetown neighborhood.

In 1928 a ballot measure was passed to construct a hospital for the "indigent sick, injured and maternity cases" on what was then known as "Profanity Hill" on the site of the former King County Courthouse and jail. This hill got its name from the 100 slippery-when-wet steep wooden stairs connecting downtown Seattle to the courthouse and so nicknamed because of the loud complaints heard from lawyers making the climb from their legal offices to court. The new hospital's location has since received the more elegant labels of First Hill and Pill Hill, so called because the area is home to medical offices and several hospitals.

Following the 1928 ballot measure, the new King County Hospital opened in 1931 as a 400-bed facility in a yellow-brick Art Deco building whose name, "Harbor View," was chosen from 6500 entries in a contest held by the *Seattle Times*. The winner, a Seattle Park Department's secretary, received the newspaper's prize of $100—about $1,600 dollars in today's currency. The old Georgetown facility, renamed King County Hospital Unit 2, served to treat patients with tuberculosis until closed and demolished in 1956.

Harborview Hall also opened in 1931. This ten-story Art Deco building, with its sleek, geometric lines and "modern" look, was constructed using the same warm beige bricks as those of the hospital. Over its entry doors are similar cast concrete, low-relief decorative panels as those placed on the hospital's main entrance. Harborview Hall housed the hospital's School of Nursing until 1961. Unused from 2011 to 2018, concerned citizens saved the building from demolition. It has since been turned into a much-needed shelter for the homeless that opened in 2018. Now, in 2020, the shelter is accessible around-the-clock. In addition to a warm, safe place to stay, this "enhanced" facility has new showers, case managers, laundry machines and a welcome for pets who are often a resident's only companion.

In 1997, two new West Hospital wings were added complementing the Art Deco style of the original structures and nearly doubling the size of the hospital. These additions are detailed with the same beige bricks and decorated with cast concrete medallions whose theme is continued on windows, doors, and stair railings in modern metal work. The buildings are occupied by clinics, offices, intensive care units, two inpatient psychiatry units, and other hospital services.

Two years later, in 1999, the Research and Training Facility opened with five laboratory floors, a vivarium, classrooms, a 150-seat auditorium, and a radiology imaging center. Of necessity, this building incorporates many technically complex mechanical and electrical systems to support these functional spaces.

All was going well until May 2019. During a planned decommissioning of a piece of medical equipment, contractors accidentally spilled a small amount of highly radioactive material. To ensure the safety of occupants and nearby personnel, the entire building was closed for the cleanup process and, as of this writing in the spring of 2020, it still remains off-limits. This has impacted the twenty medical research labs where, a month after the spill, researchers were only allowed into the building for ninety minutes to retrieve as much of their work as they could rescue.

In 2000, bond funding of $193 million was approved for the Norm Maleng Building, answering the need for seismic safety and increased space. The structure was named for former King County prosecutor Norm Maleng (1938–2007), a long-time hospital advocate whose contributions to the justice system spanned a three-decade career. Attached to the original 1931 Harborview building, this 240,000-square-foot, seventy-foot-long, six-story structure was suspended from a giant metal truss over Ninth Avenue and opened in 2008. The connecting bridge is anchored with movable pistons that will provide extra shock absorption in the event of earthquake. At night the million-pound concrete and steel walkway connecting the two buildings is illuminated by glowing cobalt-blue lights.

Along with the building's additional beds, increased space for trauma patients and operating rooms, and café that is highly praised for its special soups and made-to-order lattes, the Psychiatry Intensive Care Unit occupies the entire fifth floor. Outside of this locked unit, there are seats on the skybridge where, on nice days when "the mountain is out," trainees and their attending physicians can engage in educational interchange while enjoying a view of Mt. Rainier.

The Ninth & Jefferson Building, opened in 2009, is a fourteen-story office, clinic, and research structure located on Harborview's campus and, like other Harborview facilities, operates in partnership by King County and the University of Washington. The building houses numerous clinics and laboratories, as well as King County's medical examiner and civil commitment court. The 450,000-square-foot edifice offers stunning views of Puget Sound from its upper floors and is decorated with glorious works of art on every floor.

In the decades that followed the Harborview's opening in 1931, medical accomplishments have been numerous. In the 1940's the hospital served as treatment center for patients in the polio epidemic; Harborview established the region's first blood bank; and, in 1956, surgeons performed the West Coast's first open heart surgery. In the early 1970's the *Medic One* program was initiated to provide emergency response to those in need of life-saving care in the community and, soon afterward, the hospital became the primary training site for paramedics. Michael Copass, MD, the physician who spearheaded *Medic One*, identified the role of an air service that could transport patients distant from Seattle and so Airlift Northwest was created to carry the ill or injured to Harborview.

Today, Harborview provides a wide spectrum of services with special emphasis on trauma care and burns. It functions as the only Level 1 adult and pediatric trauma center in the four-state region. Since opening in 1974, the Regional Burn Center at Harborview has treated 20,000 patients, one-third of which are children.

The hospital's approximately 5,300 employees include 1,500 physicians, nurse practitioners and physician assistants, and 340 resident physicians-in-training. The list of provided services includes every type of surgical and medical problem imaginable, from the ordinary to the most complex and challenging.

Harborview's mission is to offer comprehensive care to patients from all walks of life, giving priority to the vulnerable or poor. In fiscal year 2018, Harborview provided more than $238 million in uncompensated care. Harborview welcomes all: immigrants, documented or otherwise; the uninsured; victims of violence; and those with mental illness and substance abuse. No one is turned away.

Working at Harborview is being a part of a community. Many employees remain at their jobs for decades, committed to the hospital's mission and feeling pride in their sense of being truly useful and necessary. When Seattle has its rare snowfall, making roads unsafe for travel, everyone in the hospital pitches in to assume tasks for snow-bound workers and do whatever is needed so that patient care continues uninterrupted.

When Seattle's 2001 earthquake struck, the hospital emptied out. People rallied outside. Somehow cups of coffee were passed around and those with phones offered to make calls for those who had none to ask about the safety of relatives at home. Strangers offered comfort to the many who were frightened.

A more cheerful event occurred with August 2017's total solar eclipse. Employees took turns to gather in front of the hospital to enjoy the spectacle. Safety glasses were shared, smartphone snaps were taken, and there was an air of a community festivity until darkness lifted, the sun returned, and everyone went inside to resume work.

As this chapter is being written at the height of the COVID19 pandemic, Harborview and its Department of Psychiatry continues to work as a system, ready to help its own and the entire community.

Harborview will remain an integral part of the local area and surrounding regions. As a pioneer in the field of medicine and a model of excellent patient care, its contributions make it a staple of the health and well-being of Seattle and the Pacific Northwest.

2

Psychiatry at Harborview

INPATIENT

When King County Hospital was renamed Harborview and opened in 1931, the fifth floor was the site of an inpatient psychiatry unit, a location remaining unchanged for eighty years. Of its patients and staff, scant records remain. No psychiatrists or nurses are still living to share memories and anecdotes of their time at work.

A single news story, appearing in the *Seattle Daily Times* on April 7, two months after the hospital's opening, gives a hint of problems in early years.

> *"Marjorie McLeod, 17-year-old patient, ...last Monday night broke through supposedly unbreakable glass and hung perilously out the window five stories above the street..."*

A county commissioner accompanied the physician as he interviewed the patient. The physician reported:

"I found no sign of insanity whatsoever. Nothing but ungovernable temper... She climbed out of the window simply to cause her guards' hearts to skip a beat or two. She succeeded—and was well pleased.

Judge Smith reiterated that if a 110-pound girl of no very great strength could force open a glass window, a violently insane person might readily do it, too...and commit suicide."

In commenting on the case, Superior Court Judge Everett Smith advised placing bars upon all windows of the psychiatric ward. The article continued:

"Acting on the suggestion of Judge Smith, the County Board of Commissioners (declined the proposal but nonetheless) ordered a fine wire mesh to be placed over windows in the psychiatric ward of Harborview Hospital."

History's documentation resumes in the 1970s with the aid of the memories of those who staffed inpatient psychiatry. David Dunner, MD, was an enthusiastic, successful, and well-trained academic who worked at the National Institute of Mental Health before becoming Harborview's Chief of Psychiatry in 1979. He recognized the need for change in management of the three inpatient units: 5 Center—the locked, intensive care unit; 8 Center—the ward housing both involuntarily detained and patients who, on their own, chose to be treated; and 3 Mental Health—the area accepting voluntary patients, situated across the street from the hospital in the freestanding mental health center.

On assuming his job, he found a demoralized faculty and a psychiatric department that had a poor public image, possibly attributed to the high turnover of patients who, after hospitalization, were returned to wander the streets with the same degree of mental illness they suffered when first admitted. To address the problem of too-brief hospital stays, Dunner called on the legal system, already in place but infrequently used. The law allowed for extending the length of stay from three to fourteen days. If the patient was believed to be still not ready for discharge, physicians could file a petition to be adjudicated in mental health court, to extend hospitalization to ninety days. Dunner found that with longer treatment, patients could be discharged in a healthier state, making readmission less likely.

Demoralized physicians were another problem Dunner addressed. He sought experienced faculty to be inpatient psychiatrists and adjusted the balance of those who would engage in research with those who focused exclusively on clinical work. Part-time faculty were hired to permit clinician-researchers to have time away from the wards to work on their academic projects. Researchers could now be comfortably productive thereby halting the rapid turnover of staff physicians.

Dunner set the tone for improvements in inpatient care; the changes he instituted made psychiatry an integral part of the hospital community and are still in effect today. His daily rounds included visits to the emergency department and consult service, and he fostered a productive relationship with representatives of the National Alliance for the Mentally Ill.

Dunner set the stage for today's successful and efficiently run three inpatient units at Harborview, housing sixty-six patients and staffed by physicians and nurses who often remain for their entire careers. Space is limited so there are no individual physician offices on site. The eight psychiatrists working on the inpatient units share a room, affectionately called the "Doctors' Dungeon," where they can consult each other for advice on puzzling cases, drink coffee, and share news of their medical and non-medical lives.

OUTPATIENT

The Community Mental Health Act of 1963, signed into law by President John F. Kennedy, provided federal funding for 1,500 community mental health centers nationwide. This act gave grants to states for the construction of facilities specially designed for the delivery of five services: mental health consultation and education; inpatient and outpatient care; emergency evaluation; and partial hospitalization. Harborview was one of the institutions benefitting from this act.

Harborview's Community Mental Health Center (HCMHC) had its beginnings in an old apartment building a few blocks from the hospital. With walk-in and crisis clinics, this service was launched with the enthusiasm and energy of psychiatrist Lindbergh Sata (1928–2006). Sata, an Asian-American physician who had survived detainment in a Japanese internment camp, became a moving force in establishing a multicultural system from what he found as the existing mono-cultural, Caucasian-based structure. He advocated for ethnic-specific mental health services after recognizing that the dropout rate was excessively high for Washington state mental health patients. Out of this era's social activism, Asian Counseling and Referral Services was founded in 1973 from a grassroots effort and with Sata's support. This organization is going strong today in providing a wide range of services, primarily for those who are low-income, immigrants, and refugees. Sata left Seattle to chair Psychiatry at St. Louis University from 1978 to 1994.

In the years that followed, HCMHC moved to its own building, a four-story brick structure on the corner of Ninth Avenue and Jefferson Street where the current Norm Maleng Building is now located. Services included a walk-in clinic, a crisis clinic, patient activity areas, rooms for therapy groups, staff offices and, on the third floor, an inpatient unit for voluntary patients. An attempt at establishing a day hospital was short-lived. This original structure was demolished to make way for the large, new, multi-purposed building. The inpatient unit, 3MH, moved to the newly constructed West Hospital wing and, in 2004, outpatient mental health relocated to the new Patricia Bracelin Steel Building named in honor of Steel (1945–2002). Her career began as a psychiatric social worker with juvenile court and, on account of her leadership skills, continued on a trajectory of serving King County government until her death.

Located three blocks from the hospital, HCMHC is now Harborview Mental Health and Addictions Services. Here, patients are offered crisis intervention, psychiatric evaluation, psychotherapy, group treatment, case management, supported employment and housing services, medication management, suicide prevention, and geriatric psychiatry services; treatment for individuals with co-occurring chemical dependency and mental health disorders; and providing care for patients with comorbid medical issues.

Psychiatry at Harborview has had a long history, with key players making critical changes to the benefit of the department. As time marches on, Psychiatry will continue to serve its diverse population of patients and will remain a force in delivery of mental health services in Seattle and surrounding areas.

3

Psychiatry's Chief of Service

With a contribution by Mark Snowden, MD, MPH

Harborview's Psychiatry and Behavioral Health Services is an important component of the University of Washington's Department of Psychiatry. One quarter of this department's 1,000 faculty, staff, and trainees serving the five-state northwest region are based at Harborview. Leading this team is its current Chief of Service, Mark Snowden.

Snowden has been a part of Harborview Psychiatry since joining the faculty in 1996.

Prior to assuming his position as Chief, he was Medical Director of Geriatric Psychiatry and Medical Director of Harborview Mental Health Services. He sees his current work as satisfying and challenging as he supports his team of psychiatrists, professionals he relies on to manage the daily tasks of running the inpatient and outpatient hospital and clinic services. As Chief, he is available for advice and action when needed, and, by taking this approach, he remains free to devote his time to interfacing with administration and participating in strategic planning for the hospital and his service.

Situations requiring immediate attention can arise unexpectedly, and thus, providers are encouraged to contact Snowden for advice whether it is confronting a difficulty involving an individual patient or requesting help in negotiating a sometimes-unwieldy system. In a place as busy as Harborview, unpredicted crises can occur, and when no one knows exactly what to do in those moments. Snowden helps to find a solution.

Sometimes answers are not easily found, however. To maintain the department's aim to offer inpatient care to the many who need it, an ideal resolution was thought to reopen a previously closed psychiatric unit only for Snowden to learn that it was impossible: The plumbing in this aging building was irrevocably clogged.

Snowden has received calls asking for help from unexpected locations. He was contacted by an outside clinic who told him that a patient was in their waiting room who had been detained while on Harborview's Consult Service. A family member had encouraged their relative to leave the hospital so that he could be taken to this health center for care. Since the patient was neither discharged nor was he ready to leave, Snowden organized an administrative team who drove to the clinic to escort the patient back to Harborview.

Approximately forty psychiatrists along with a number of psychologists, physician assistants, and nurse practitioners comprise Harborview's roster of providers. Psychiatrists are generally pleased and proud to be part of this hospital's mission and community and, once starting work, often remain with the institution for decades. Others, with no one to blame, decide to depart after only a few years' work. These physicians will have their own reasons for leaving: the opportunity for higher earnings elsewhere, the need to be in a different city to accommodate family obligations, or the pressure created by the demand to sign a non-compete document that bars the provider from practicing within a ten-mile radius for two years after leaving a university facility and can be enforced by law. Recognizing the shortage of psychiatrists, this restriction has been now been reduced.

The present situation in terms of providers, physical space, and the daily workings of Psychiatry at Harborview is stable. Many changes are in progress for the rest of the department, but there has been no urgency to consider major adjustments at this facility, but more space would always be enthusiastically welcomed for outpatient care and to expand research and training programs. The developing University of Washington Behavioral Health Institute will be located at Harborview, as it supports the largest clinical and training program within the Department of Psychiatry and Behavioral Sciences. Its purpose will be to create innovative activities and to support faculty and staff as they strive to improve care and experience for patients with behavioral health issues. Plans are in progress to establish access for teens and young adults experiencing their first episode of psychosis, to expand regional telepsychiatry options and to strengthen current crisis intervention services.

Snowden heads a very active Quality Improvement (QI) program, advanced in its design and management. Meetings attended by a dozen or more representatives of the service—nurses, physicians, social workers, and administrators—occur twice a month. Here, problems arising from untoward patient events are examined and reviewed as to how they were handled and what can be done, if at all possible, to avoid similar events in the future. Another aspect of the QI meeting is to identify various metrics and discuss the results with an aim to ultimately improve the already-high caliber of psychiatric treatment Harborview provides.

The QI program tracks measures associated with patient care. The committee looks at patients' ease of access to medical attention. For example, they review the time it takes from a patient presenting in the Psychiatric Emergency Service to the moment when a provider greets them and begins their evaluation. Time is also measured from completion of the provider's assessment to the arrival of the Designated Crisis Responder (DCR), a Washington state-trained mental health professional, who determines if hospital admission is warranted. This neutral, county-employed professional interviews the patient and weighs collateral evidence to decide if the patient is a danger to themselves or others or they cannot care for their own health and safety. If, after careful consideration, the DCR concludes that inpatient hospitalizaton is indicated, metrics track the amount of time from assessment to admission.

Other metrics are monitored in both in- and outpatient settings. Of note is that Psychiatry is unique as being the only hospital service that measures timeliness of response to consult requests with the goal of seeing 75% of patients within ninety minutes of telephone referral. In the outpatient Mental Health Center, metrics record the length of time elapsing between the request for an initial appointment and when it appears on the schedule. Additionally, metrics document how much time elapses before the patient can be seen for the second follow-up visit.

Long before measurements were required, Harborview began its own assessment of whether psychiatric medicines produced side effects referred to as the "metabolic syndrome." If not closely monitored, patients are at risk for developing diabetes, high blood pressure, and excessive weight gain as a result of taking certain medications.

Metrics are also called up to reflect staff satisfaction, but the ultimate goal is to show that Harborview Psychiatry quantitatively provides the best care to every single person, even when other facilities might turn them away.

4

Psychiatry Emergency Service

With contributions by Paul Borghesani, MD, PhD;
Christos Dagadakis, MD; Craig Jaffe, MD;
Hannah McCluskey, RN-BC, BSN; and
Jennifer Schmitt, RN, BSN, CCRN

Dedicated psychiatric emergency services (PES) are now recognized as an important and much-needed resource, and from the time the first emergency department (ED) opened its doors, it became obvious that patients with psychiatric conditions required special care. Although many psychiatric services exist today in various forms, their development is still in progress.

The origins of today's PES are found in the regular EDs, now ubiquitous in the US and around the world. The specialty of emergency medicine received recognition in the 1960s then gained official status in 1979. Yet EDs are currently taxed to the limits of their capacity. In 2017, they treated 145.6 million patients across the country, and 4.5% of all ED visits are attributed to mental health problems, including substance abuse, suicidal or violent thoughts, and psychosis. With constantly increasing demand, a specialized area, the PES, was established to meet the growing need for dedicated mental health evaluations and care. By 1971, dedicated services were available in about 1,000 general and psychiatric hospitals in the US. A rising number of patients now are treated in these specialized hospital units.

Harborview Medical Center (HMC) saw its service established in 1983 at the inspiration of a working psychiatrist, Dr. Christos Dagadakis. From the beginning, there was resentment from the regular ED with competition for space, a situation that has persisted with more or less fervor, for decades. The current arrangement for the PES took about ten years of planning to put into place. Multiple consultants were called upon to help justify the amount of space requested. Separated by locked doors from the rest of the ED, the PES treats an impressive number of psychiatric patients: Over 4,000 individuals were evaluated from October 2018 to November 2019, averaging 333 visits a month.

The original HMC PES recruited social workers to assess patients with mental health needs. These specialists organized and led the PES team with only a part-time physician presence. Even today, it is often the social worker in many general emergency facilities who initiate evaluation of patients with mental health concerns.

As a rule, psychiatrists do not staff emergency departments in most hospitals in the US. Only large urban or academic centers have full-time specialists. At Harborview, seventeen doctors work part- or full-time and cover each shift around the clock. In addition, there are nurse practitioners and two or three registered nurses along with several mental health professionals: men and women without a nursing degree but highly trained to care for the needs and behaviors of the mentally ill. Completing the treatment team is the shift's social worker. All staff are trained in de-escalation techniques designed to defuse potentially tense or violent situations, including specific skills such as how to listen without being condescending or dismissive, and how to restrain patients gently, a procedure needed to reduce agitation and avoid violence. When a person is sufficiently agitated to put staff at risk for harm, security officers arrive within moments of an urgent call.

Whether arriving on their own or brought by family, police, or friends, the ED's triage nurse may decide that initial medical screening is needed. If the problem is mainly psychiatric, and if one of the nine PES beds is available, the nurse escorts them to this specialized unit. If a bed is unavailable but the person is calm, they remain in the general waiting area. Unstable patients are taken to the main ED to await the psychiatric team's visit. Violent or actively suicidal individuals may be restrained to prevent harm to themselves, staff, or others. Not infrequently, the PES plus the ED evaluate up to twenty patients at a time with mental health concerns.

Once within the secure PES area, the patient is taken to one of nine separate rooms. Each can be locked if necessary for safety, and all are video monitored. The environment's design is to provide a soothing, neutral space that reduces stimulation. There are no windows, and the furniture consists of a bed and plastic chair. Lighting is low. Many arrive excited and disorganized and in need of calm. Patients receive three meals a day plus snacks and beverages on request. Staff obtain basic laboratory studies to screen for immediate medical problems. Tests include blood studies and a urinalysis to assess for kidney or urine abnormality. The urine is also tested for the presence of illegal drugs such as methamphetamine and opioids as well as for marijuana, a substance legal in Washington state but still one that can distort the patient's thinking and induce irrational behaviors.

Patients may seek treatment for mental health issues on their own or perhaps their friends, family, or care provider have encouraged them to do so. About a third of those in the PES voluntarily ask for help with their depression, are troubled by hearing voices, recognize that their substance use disorder is out of control, or they just arrive seeking a refill for their psychiatric medication.

Police find individuals on the street behaving in a disruptive, threatening, or bizarre manner and bring them to the hospital. Such persons generally don't want to be evaluated or cared for and are resistant to attempts to engage them. A physician who works in the King County Jail and in the PES describes how often he sees patients whom he recognizes from both facilities. He comments that both systems are imperfect but takes pride in his work, recognizing that "we're the ones that catch them as they're falling and try to set them on the right track. We can give medical and psychiatric care for problems they themselves don't admit to having."

One physician describes how he tries to help patients who don't want to be in the PES:

> "I try to help them figure out why they were brought here. I tell them I understand that they don't want to be here but as long as they're stuck, what can we work on to make things better? I ask them what needs to happen so that you can leave? I tell them I'm here to help you resume your life. Let's work on this together. As long as someone's not spitting and fighting, we can have a conversation and find some common ground and figure out something productive."

A final group of patients are referred by community providers who see dangerous or unusual behaviors. If the patient dwells on the notion of suicide or make clear threats to harm themselves, the provider then decides that it is unsafe for the person to remain outside of the hospital. A person might divulge a plan, no matter how vague, to physically harm someone else and that, too is cause to send them to the PES. The patient may try to convince their provider that they're safe and willing go to the hospital on their own but, if suspicious, the clinician calls the police to escort the person directly to the hospital, ensuring safe arrival in the PES before any harm is done.

Conditions treated in the PES are serious. Gone are the days when life difficulties or feeling somewhat depressed justify a request for hospitalization for psychotherapy. Contrary to a misconception of the providers' mission in the PES, their role is not just to counsel people who are sad or to provide temporary support. Today's patients who are considered for hospitalization are far more disturbed than those seen in the outpatient setting.

Suicidal thoughts are sufficient reason for PES evaluation. A person may have passive thoughts of death or suffer from a profound depression and are determined to take their own life. They may have a definite plan to shoot or hang themselves or set a situation to incite the police to shoot them. They may have a stockpile of their own pills either prescribed or obtained from others as a ready means to die. Or they might have identified the bridge or highway overpass from which they will jump. Patients can create imaginative means to end their lives.

A 29-year-old man with a history of heavy marijuana use decided that he no longer wanted to live after his girlfriend ended their relationship. He drove to a freeway overpass, stopped his car, rushed to the railing, and jumped. His body came crashing down on the roof of an SUV driven by an 80-year-old retired professor on his way to a woodcarving class. The elderly man suffered a fractured neck in addition to multiple other injuries and the young man who jumped also had fractures and a ruptured spleen.

Both men were taken to Harborview. By coincidence, they were placed in opposite beds in the Intensive Care Unit. Miraculously, both survived and the elderly man has gone on to continue his pursuit of woodcarving.

Thoughts to harm or kill another absolutely require attention. A person may have a plan, driven by paranoia or other delusions, that someone either directly known to them or perhaps even a stranger is going to harm them, making them believe that they must kill first for self- protection. Patients can be angry and want to injure people they know or may feel homicidal toward others in general. They might, or might not, admit to having a weapon or reveal that they know exactly where to get one. Homicidal rage is a common reason for a PES evaluation.

On occasion, children are brought to the PES. A nurse recalls a memorable experience with a potentially homicidal child:

"I received a call informing me that an ambulance service had brought a 6-year-old boy who needed an emergency psychiatric evaluation. This child had been in the care of his 12-year-old sister while his mother attended a community college night class. The girl was tormenting her brother, and he'd had as much as any child could bear so he grabbed a knife from the kitchen, chased his sister and yelled that he meant to stab her.

Escaping, the girl locked herself in the bathroom and called 911. The police arrived and took the 6-year-old to the PES, a place that can be quite scary even for the most seasoned adult.

I was struck by how small he looked sitting on an adult-sized stretcher. The little boy told me that he really didn't want to kill his sister but couldn't figure out another way to make the torment stop. Tearful and frightened, he just wanted his mom. I got him some coloring books. After talking to our psychiatrist, social worker, and a member of the Children's Crisis Outreach Response Team (CCORS), everyone decided that it was safe for the child to go home with his mother's promise to make an alternative arrangement for childcare."

Finally, it may be obvious that a person cannot care for themselves. They may be troubled by hearing voices, believe that others are going to harm them, or are in other ways disconnected from reality. Individuals living on the street are not necessarily candidates for hospitalization; however, if mental illness makes existence precarious and persons are unable to obtain food or medicines, are in obvious need of medical care, or are infested with parasites, the social and medical system is obliged to step in and evaluate their ability to make choices for self-care. Washington state law permits commitment to a hospital for a gravely disabled patient.

Patients often arrive in the PES intoxicated with alcohol, marijuana, or illegal substances. Drugs go in and out of fashion. Today's choice psychotropic substance is methamphetamine while at other times crack cocaine or heroin were in vogue. Several thousand patients each year present with the psychosis and violence accompanying methamphetamine intoxication. Hallucinogens including mushrooms and LSD have had their periods of popularity while designer drugs such as bath salts and ecstasy still make an occasional appearance. Cocaine abuse is fairly common with its subsequent dysphoria, depression, and suicidal thoughts. Opiates can be taken in large enough quantity to cause an acute overdose, but this is a medical emergency treated by medical colleagues. Fewer alcohol intoxications are seen in recent years because of the availability of sobering centers and detoxification facilities so patients can bypass the ED for treatment.

Marijuana, legal in Washington state, is a drug that many patients use daily; the urine screen for cannabis is positive for more than half of those evaluated in the PES. Over the past five years it's been firmly established that marijuana can unmask dormant mental illness or inflame an already existing mania or psychosis. Marijuana is especially toxic in its man-made highly concentrated form: "Dabs" is condensed THC oil prepared to be smoked and whose subsequently wild psychotic symptoms can last for weeks.

It's indisputable that anyone with a mental health diagnosis— from anxiety to depression to schizophrenia—should not be using marijuana. A considerable fraction of cases of new-onset psychosis that resemble schizophrenia can be attributed to high potency cannabis use. Here in Seattle, THC, the active compound of cannabis, is rising in concentration in the marijuana available for purchase. The average content in cities like Amsterdam and Copenhagen is 10% in commercially sold products while it is 20% in those sold in Seattle.

While intoxicated, a person cannot coherently participate in an evaluation. In a general ED, assessment begins within minutes of arrival, but the time course is different for those who arrive in the PES under the influence of a legal or illegal substance. They are allowed to sleep for as long as it takes for their body to metabolize the drug. After several to as many as twenty-four hours, the person can be deemed sober enough to allow the provider to proceed with the interview. While waiting, clinicians review the accompanying police report and gather collateral information from those who are familiar with the patient.

Each person in the PES is treated with respect and dignity. The patient is first greeted by a nurse, physician, or medical student, then is escorted to their room. Sitting on their bed, a nurse or nursing technician checks blood pressure, pulse, and temperature. If staff find a significant abnormality, the physician confers with their counterpart in the regular medical ED. If necessary, the patient is transferred to the ED or, if there is no indication of a medical problem requiring immediate care, the psychiatric evaluation proceeds. The first task is to establish rapport. The patient is asked the reason for the visit and is encouraged to tell their story of recent events. The clinician gathers information about their past psychiatric and social history as well as current medications and treatment. The aim is to make a temporary diagnosis and plan the best course of action to help with the current situation.

There are times when a patient can be put on the right course for help to the relief of an anxious family. One PES physician recalls:

"A family brought their aging relative to the PES. He'd had a long history of working in his own food business but now, at 80, looking like he had a form of Parkinson's disease, he was horribly depressed. He'd been at another hospital where he was vaguely suicidal but was sent home with an antidepressant medicine and advice to return if he felt worse. His wife and daughter were dissatisfied and troubled by this treatment. As depression increased and he began to speak more about wanting to end his life, his family brought him to Harborview.

The gentleman agreed to enter the hospital where, thankfully, a bed was open for him. His loving and concerned family were pleased that he would not only get needed psychiatric care but that there would be a geriatric medical specialist and a neurologist to address all of his many medical needs."

Behaviors can raise friends' concern. For example, a college student, although reluctant, was convinced to accompany his roommates to the PES because he'd been missing classes, not sleeping, speaking too rapidly and, at times, yelling and not making sense. Mania is a common reason for a PES evaluation.

Many patients will describe their troubles, but others may decide to refuse to talk. Everyone has the right to be silent but that makes an assessment of the situation more difficult. According to law, the social worker is permitted to call family members, outside care providers, or even friends to try to flesh out the story of what is now going on and how the PES can help.

Safety is foremost. A suicidal or homicidal person can attempt to act on impulse, as do patients who are agitated and violent for myriad reasons. Prevention is imperative. Sometimes talking alone is helpful. A feeling of being listened to can go a long way. If necessary, trained security guards are called upon to maintain safety by placing them in seclusion or even physical restraints.

Patients receive medicine when they are anxious or so troubled that they lose control of their words or actions. Drugs are chosen from a general class of sedatives, the benzodiazepines or, if they have also lost touch with reality, they receive an antipsychotic. It is first offered by mouth or, if it is deemed necessary by their level of distress, drugs are administered by injection.

Medicines are also prescribed for other reasons such as to make up for a dose missed at home. If a patient complains of severe itching and, like some homeless clients, scabies, bed bugs, or lice are found, treatment starts with pills and shampoo.

Many severely mentally ill patients have a miscellany of medical illnesses. Some are conditions also found in a general population like diabetes, hypertension, and HIV infection. Patients with HIV are often in various stages of therapy, but some have been refusing treatment. Other rarer ailments are seen in the homeless who stay in shelters or sleep outside, such as tuberculosis, untreated wounds, and parasite infestations. PES providers diagnose and initiate treatment and set a plan for follow-up when possible.

After evaluation, clinicians decide on the next step for care. If it is deemed safe for the patient to leave the hospital, the social worker can arrange for transportation then a return to their outpatient clinic or obtain an appointment in Harborview outpatient services. Sadly, many have no interest in follow-up and neglect to keep their appointments. It becomes yet more difficult if they have no established care and no home to return to. There are limited options for patients ready to leave the PES but not ready to return to the street. Unfortunately, there are only a few respite beds or crisis centers offering shelter for those who may need it most. Sadly, though, an unclean and crowded shelter or discharge to the street may be the only option.

Washington state's rules on who must be detained to hospital are firm. If a person is a definite danger to themselves or to others or they are considered so gravely disabled that they cannot provide for their own food and well-being, they can be hospitalized against their will. Of course, this is not as easy as said. There are usually a lmited number of available beds at Harborview or in the regional hospitals for the social worker to secure. Until obtaining a bed is feasible, the patient will "board" in the PES, for hours or sometimes for days. There is medication and food but no actual psychiatric treatment other than maintaining a holding pattern of safety. This is a universally problematic situation that worsens as time goes by.

Staffing the PES is not easy. This service must be covered around the clock, yet, if given the choice, physicians prefer not to work evenings and nights; social workers and nurses are also reluctant to agree to fill these shifts. Further, there is always the risk of assault. Arrest is often a possibility but the decision to call the police is made on a case-by-case assessment and is one that providers often struggle with. Many patients have both mental health concerns and a long history of legal issues as well. True, jail provides mental health care, but this option may not be in the patient's best interest. For example, an elderly man with dementia, brought in by his family because he is assaulting them, certainly would not be better served if incarcerated rather than hospitalized.

Violence can impact even a 6'2" powerful-appearing physician who recalls a frightening incident:

> "A man was brought in by a family member concerned that his relative had lost touch with reality. The patient was muttering unintelligibly. "I began to ask him what was troubling him, but he didn't answer my question but began to say 'Your eyes, your eyes' and with outstretched fingers reached out to grab my face. I usually wear glasses but had my contacts in and that made it even scarier."

The PES is a high-stress job for all who work there. Physicians and staff must confront patients when intoxicated, psychotic, cognitively impaired by dementia or developmental delay, and not yet medicated. In spite of the risk of physical harm, those who work in the PES do so with a sense of pride that they are on the front line of mental health care and are starting patients on the best possible path to treatment and recovery.

5

Social Work in the Psychiatric Emergency Service

With a contribution by Nicole Blythe, MSW

The social worker, a vital member of the Psychiatric Emergency Service (PES) team, may be the first provider to meet the patient after they've been welcomed and settled in by nursing staff. As in other psychiatric services, the social worker is viewed as the person who offers help and comfort to a distressed person who may not want to be in the hospital at all and, unlike the medical team, doesn't order unwanted or disagreeable medications.

The social worker gives the patient the opportunity to share their story in a safe space. They, like all staff and providers, give assurance that they will be heard and not judged. Patients are encouraged to speak about whatever is on their mind and describe events prior to coming to emergency services whether by their own choice or by someone else's insistence. They receive no criticism for substance abuse or for untoward behaviors. The social worker affirms that they are there to help.

Safety is a primary concern for all patients and especially for those who are possible victims of abuse. The social worker asks direct questions which the person may choose to answer or not but, in their best interest, the inquiry must be made, such as: Do you feel safe going home? Do you want to call the police? If the individual is over eighteen years old, they get to choose if they want to return to their residence or feel the need to find a safe, temporary place away from the abuser by seeking the protection of a relative or a domestic violence shelter. If minors are at home, laws are called into action to protect children as well as pets because an aggressor may be threatening to harm animals in the house.

If the victim of domestic violence is cleared by PES providers to leave, they may still want to return home even though professionals advise that this choice is unsafe. The social worker makes sure that a victim has the resources on hand to support escape should that become necessary. If they have to run in the middle of the night, they will know who to call and where to go in those critical moments of attempting to elude an assailant. Should written material accompany the victim? Would it be more of a problem if the abuser finds brochures on domestic violence and uses the discovery as a reason for revenge? The social worker and victim discuss where to hide materials so that they are available if needed.

Elder abuse is a growing problem in our aging population. Patients in the PES, even though subject to physical or emotional abuse by the relatives who care for them, are often reluctant to disclose their experience because of a sense of shame. If there is direct evidence of physical harm such as bruises in unexpected locations or injuries cause by an unexplained fall, the social worker asks if the patient would like to have the police notified. If the person declines, and they are intent on returning home after discharge, a safety plan is put in place. If the elder is extremely vulnerable or is disabled, the social worker considers making a referral to Adult Protective Services or to police and let the law take its course.

Ronald, a 78-year-old man with early dementia, was brought to the PES by police. His neighbor was concerned when he saw Ronald in his yard, appearing dirty and looking confused. The neighbor observed him only going in and out of the garden shed and never into or out of his house.

The police found Ronald confined to the shed, surrounded by trash and rotten food. They discovered that Ronald's daughter put him there, forbidding him to enter the house. The daughter was exploiting Ronald's resources and draining his bank account. She was known to the police as a methamphetamine user.

Adult Protective Services was called by the PES social worker. Ronald was admitted to the Psychiatric Intensive Care Unit rather than to a less restrictive setting, as he was intent on escaping from the hospital to return to his daughter. Placement was an issue since Ronald refused to go to an adult family home or any other option. He was on the wait list for the dementia unit at Western State Hospital and had to remain at Harborview for many months until a bed became available. Even though there was a protection order forbidding contact with his daughter, he would ask almost daily to be allowed to return to live with her. Yet, when he was able to be transferred to the next facility, he did so with an unexpected display of appreciation for the staff who had so attentively cared for him.

The Center for Disease Control reports that nearly 1 in 5 women and 1 in 38 men have experienced completed or attempted rape. Those who rely on Harborview for care are trying to manage significant mental health troubles and are often especially vulnerable to sexual predators. In the PES they may speak about abuse that occurred as a child but also may reveal that they have been recently assaulted. The social worker then initiates an important cascade of events.

The patient is taken to the main Emergency Department (ED) for a physical examination. An on-call nurse, specially trained at Harborview's Abuse & Trauma Center, conducts a forensic examination, offers treatment for a possible sexually transmitted infection, and provides emergency contraception. It is important for a victim to feel sufficiently safe and cared for by someone who understands the nature of their traumatic experience. This care is no guarantee to prevent the possible consequences of assault—depression, acute- or post-traumatic stress disorder, and even thoughts of suicide—but initial understanding and support can only sound a positive note as the person moves forward.

On leaving the PES, the social worker creates a safe follow-up plan. There is a referral to Harborview's special trauma clinic where brief counselling is offered to victims of rape. Sadly, there are at least several patients a week who are evaluated in the PES for sexual assault.

Arranging for care for all patients after discharge from the PES is a social work challenge. There are a few, but far from many, alternatives to psychiatric hospitalization. The Crisis Solutions Center is a nationally recognized provider to homeless and vulnerable mentally ill individuals. One component is the Crisis Diversion Facility, a sixteen-bed residential treatment program. It is a small, freestanding structure where patients can be feels safe as they stay for three days of care. Here they receive mental health and chemical dependence assessments and intensive case management. Eligibility for this option means being in good behavioral control and not having committed a violent crime.

Another option is the twenty-bed Crisis Respite Program in downtown Seattle that offers a month of a stable setting with mental health support. Patients are not confined to the facility and can leave to keep appointments or just go for a walk. This program serves as a buffer between psychiatric emergency care and return to the streets, providing links to medical and psychiatric services and the important initiation of the search for housing.

Many patients evaluated in the PES need immediate attention to their substance use and addiction. Two medical detoxification facilities in King County accept Washington state insurance and can help people struggling with alcohol and illegal substances. Participation is voluntary. The person is referred from the PES to the ED for medical clearance to look for existing conditions that might make it unsafe to undergo immediate detoxification. If approved, the social worker calls the detox facility, which does a telephone screening. This process may take several hours of coordination with many people involved but, hopefully, acceptance for treatment occurs on the same day. Once there, the patient is referred to chemical dependency services such as a counselor or case manager for continued support.

Another time-consuming task is identifying a hospital to care for someone needing inpatient treatment when Harborview has no bed available. Multiple requests and long waits for return calls can make this a thankless endeavor with no guarantee of success.

In spite of stress and demands, the social worker, with kindness and patience, gives comfort and support to patients and their families and serves as an indispensable member of the treatment team.

6

The Psychiatric Intensive Care Unit

When first stepping into the Psychiatric Intensive Care Unit (ICU), the atmosphere of calm can be remarkably deceptive. The light green and pale-yellow walls are accented by bland, industrial carpeting or tan textured tiles. Posters of artwork, maps, and photography hang on the walls. Monet's *Water Lilies* and an inviting photograph of a bridge in Venice add to the ambience.

This environment is actually far from serene. Because of the potentially violent patient population, everything must be designed for safety. You get a hint when you realize that the posters are mounted behind thick acrylic plates bolted to the wall. Furniture is large and simple. Each of the primary-colored chairs can weigh as much as seventy-five pounds to prevent being them from being picked up and thrown as a weapon. Dining tables in the dayroom are bolted to the floor, as are the base of the swiveling chairs. At times, there's a hole in the wall covered temporarily by plastic. This could have been made by a patient punching in a fit of rage and now the carpenters are awaited to make repairs.

Patient rooms are pleasant but bare, as they lack the decorations and amenities usually found in a general hospital room. There are no closets—these would be too tempting for a patient intent on committing suicide by hanging. For clothing and the minimal personal belongings patients bring with them, there are open shelves anchored to the wall secure enough so that a sumo wrestler with a crowbar couldn't pry them loose. There are no bedside tables, as these could be used as missiles to heave at staff. A table could also be propped against the door as an obstruction, preventing access to a patient committing an act of self-harm. The bed is also secured to the floor to prevent it from becoming a weapon or barricade. Likewise, a secured bedframe cannot move if the patient is restrained against their intentional or inadvertent movements to harm themselves or others.

Bathrooms are spartan as well. No curtains or glass enclosure on the shower that drains to the floor. And even with a strainer covering the drainpipe to prevent objects from clogging it, patients can still set towels on the shower floor to flood the bathroom. Toilets are no exception: plugged with clothing or whatever paper is at hand, staff must rapidly place an emergency call to Environmental Services when patients sabotage the plumbing.

The unit has twenty-one private rooms that never go unoccupied. Patients needing intensive care who cannot be maintained safely on another unit may have to wait for an available bed for several days in the emergency area. Once admitted to the ICU, a person will have a clean, pleasant space; some look out on an impressive view of Puget Sound with its boats, barges, and skyline.

Safeguarding patients and those who care for them are foremost. To prevent an individual jumping through glass to land five floors below, all windows are covered with a heavy mesh protective screen whose integrity is verified by staff's frequent security checks.

The unit is laid out in the shape of a "U." Although halls are monitored by staff and cameras, there would remain a considerable escape risk through doors partially hidden around a corner so exits at either end have been disabled. Before permanent decommissioning, a heavily pregnant and psychotic patient flung her body against this securely locked door, broke through, and escaped. Security was alerted and she was returned to the unit. After a repeat of the same forceful exit, the door was permanently sealed, and now the only one route of entry and exit is accessed by visitors: a telephone. If a patient is intent on escape and flee through the single interior door they must traverse a long hallway to the exterior door, giving staff an opportunity to confine them before they can leave the unit.

Patients who test door handles and post themselves by the entryway, necessitate "escape precautions": their shoes are replaced by non-slip socks. Wearing a hospital gown and robe rather than street clothing also serves as a technique of discouraging the potential escapee from trying to leave the hospital. If a patient does accomplish a successful exit—as did one patient who hid in a laundry cart, then quietly wheeled off the unit without attracting attention —hospital security and police are notified to find and return the person to complete the hospitalization for which they have been legally committed.

Although minimal, patients have basic entertainments. Art and music groups are led by staff. Two television sets, one on either end of the dayroom and secured to the wall by heavy bolts, offer a limited choice of channels. TV stations with violent and provocative content are unavailable so viewing is limited to news, cartoons, movies, and drama and comedy shows.

Those confined to the hospital have access to other media and activities. A radio can be locked behind the metal window screen and staff changes stations at the patient's request. One of the two conference rooms features a DVD player for movies and a ping pong table—which is only rarely used, as patients are often too disorganized to engage in a game. The other meeting room has a sadly off-pitch piano, donated several years ago and only tuned on occasion when sufficient funds can be found to pay for the services of piano technician to work on the instrument. There's a supply of checkers, chess, board games, and puzzles. Telephones are available for use during daytime and evening hours, but telephone privileges are withheld from patients who harass others. Patients who call 911 and ask for the police to come and release them from the unit are also kept from using the phone until they can agree to stop making these calls. Internet access isn't provided on the ICU, but staff is willing to do a search when requested.

Food is plentiful. Each patient is given a menu with the next day's choices; if he or she has difficulty choosing or understanding, staff offers assistance. Food quality is excellent with substantial portions attractively prepared. Caffeinated coffee is served only once in the morning. Excess caffeine for patients already experiencing the adrenaline surge of agitation caused by mental illness is contraindicated but cups of decaf are at hand. Snacks of toasted cheese sandwiches, fruit, and yogurt are served several times throughout the day and evening. A patient who has difficulty sleeping and craves something to eat during the night is given a choice of food items to calm and comfort.

Patients receive standard medical care. Consultants from all medical and surgical specialties offer their expertise. Because about a third to half of the twenty-one patients in the ICU also have compounding medical conditions, many beds are regular hospital equipment that change as needed in position and height. All treatments are rendered similar to those provided throughout the hospital including IVs and oxygen. Portable x-rays are ordered if the patient is too ill or uncooperative to travel to the x-ray department. An electrocardiogram machine, a blood pressure reading device, and an apparatus that measures oxygen saturation of the blood is readily available. Laboratory technicians come to the unit at any time to draw blood if the floor nurse is unable to do so. If a patient has a medical emergency, staff calls the team of specialized nurses and the response is immediate, then this team is quickly followed by a consultant in medicine, surgery, or other medical specialty required to administer emergency care. If needed, the patient can be transferred for continued care in a medical ICU or to a treatment floor.

As on every inpatient unit at Harborview, those hospitalized arrive with a variety of medical illnesses, some longstanding and others newly diagnosed. Many are admitted from the street or from shelters. If they've been prescribed medicine they're not taking, it might be that pills were discarded or stolen so they get medical care only through occasional emergency department (ED) visits.

Either before they arrive in the ICU or after they are settled in, all patients have laboratory studies that screen for anemia, kidney, thyroid and liver function and for an infection reflected in a blood or urine test. Evaluation for the presence of marijuana, alcohol, and drugs such as methamphetamine, cocaine, and opioids has usually been done in the Psychiatric Emergency Service (PES) or ED.

Ignored medical conditions can now be set right with evaluation and treatment. Diabetes and high blood pressure are fairly common. A person on the street is unlikely to check their blood sugar or to go to a fire station or pharmacy for a blood pressure reading. In most cases, it is easy to get the patient on the right track with finger-stick blood sugars and blood pressure checks. In order for these life-prolonging treatments such as pills and insulin to work, however, the patient must agree to take them. A return to previous unhealthy and insecure living conditions often means that the hard work of hospital physicians and nurses will be undone.

Sometimes a patient describes a new physical symptom, different from previous complaints. It's up to staff and physicians to be sufficiently alert to assess when a problem stems from emotional distress or from a true physical abnormality.

Thomas, a twenty-three-year-old man with schizophrenia, spent much of his time lying in bed, reluctant to speak with staff, other patients or even watch TV. He'd accept his antipsychotic medication but asked no questions and had little to say about them. His staff noticed that he was eating less. In fact, he was barely eating at all. When asked if he had pain, he denied feeling bad but when the vigilant nurse suggested that he touch Thomas' belly, he flinched and winced even when the nurse placed his hand lightly on his middle. Paging the physician on call, the wheels were set in motion for blood tests, a surgical consult and the result was a decision to take the patient to the operating room to remove a very diseased appendix in time to prevent a possible fatal rupture.

The story of another patient in the psychiatric ICU did not end as well but better than if he been someplace other than Harborview.

Mr. C, a thin, middle-aged man looking worn and worried, had spent most of his adult life on the street. Buying and selling cocaine was his all-consuming activity. His psychosis, fueled by drugs, could make him wild but he could be quite calm when he wasn't high.   -

   Mr. C had visited the emergency department on several occasions with complaints of abdominal discomfort and nausea but, after a brief evaluation, was usually discharged with a bottle of antacid and the admonition to stop using cocaine.

On one visit, cocaine caused Mr. C to be sufficiently delusional to warrant an admission to the psychiatric ICU. Here he was eventually calmed by medications, but his complaints of abdominal pain worsened.

A cascade of events followed. The medical consultant recommended calling the gastroenterologists. They evaluated the patient with x-rays then an endoscopy where a lighted tube was placed in the stomach to see if there was any abnormality such as an ulcer. Although ulcer was the expected finding, the unexpected was seen instead: a cancer of the stomach.

Mr. C had his surgery then returned for care in psychiatry. He stabilized then was sent to a nursing care facility. As occasionally happens, his staff and physicians liked this man from the streets and would visit him at his residence. For the first time in a very long time, Mr. C had a bed with clean linens and people who cared about him. Unfortunately, his disease rapidly progressed, and he was brought back to Harborview. In the hospital that had given him the experience of good, concerned caretakers, his life came to a peaceful end.

Patients come from a variety of backgrounds, but many are homeless or inadequately housed. Families bring their relative when they can no longer care for a person who is assaultive, destructive of property and, in general, out of control. Occasionally, an individual is brought from the airport, having arrived by plane and noted by authorities to be disruptive. Others arrive in Seattle by bus or having hitchhiked from a distant state. One patient revealed that she traveled to Seattle, lured by the prospect of legal marijuana. Some patients have ignored the psychiatric medications that might have been prescribed in a previous hospitalization in another state and they are currently struggling with the symptoms of psychosis and are intoxicated with drugs.

Harborview has been the hospital for patients from other countries. A graduate student from Brazil with no mental health history became psychotic. As part of his evaluation, a brain scan showed that he suffered from a neurologic disease causing his psychiatric symptoms. Persons from Europe and Asia, working at Seattle's high-tech companies, have had psychiatric decompensations and stayed in the psychiatric ICU until stabilized.

A twenty-four-year-old schizophrenic man found enough money for a plane ticket and, slipping away from his parents, traveled from Norway to seek a Seattle woman he'd learned about online. He was picked up by the police wandering a neighborhood north of downtown ringing doorbells in hope of finding her. Once brought to Harborview, treatment was started, and his family was contacted in Oslo. Relieved to hear that their missing son was safe, they flew to collect him in Seattle when his hospital stay was complete, bringing a selection of woolly hats and mittens in gratitude for those who had cared for their son.

All patients are welcome no matter where they are from. Everyone is equally treated with proper medications, offered clean clothing and food, and encouraged to tell their stories. Each patient is assigned a "contact person," a staff member who gives individual attention during the shift as well as a nurse who supervises medication and medical care. Not all patients want to talk. Everyone understands that there can be significant resentment at someone having to be hospitalized against their will causing a person to exercise their choice and refuse to speak.

Patients are treated for a variety of diagnoses. Most have some form of psychotic disorder like schizophrenia or substance-induced psychosis or the loss of touch with reality accompanying a version of bipolar disorder. Sadly, there are no other alternative facilities where persons with certain conditions can go. Those with developmental disabilities and autism who are too dysregulated and violent for other settings are cared for in Harborview's psychiatric ICU. They are attended to with kindness and compassion by staff. Even though this unit is not geared to treat and provide activities for patients with developmental issues, they sometimes stay for a year or more because no other placement can be found. Dedicated facilities in western Washington are closing and the appropriate unit at the state hospital is always filled to capacity. There have been times when up to a third of the twenty-one beds are occupied by patients awaiting a place to go.

It is equally difficult to find placement for dementia patients. They have been admitted to Harborview because their family or residential facility cannot manage the problems of cognitive impairment: wandering, aggression, or neglected self-care. Women with dementia, considered too vulnerable to be with the mix of psychotic and sometimes predatory males, do not stay in the ICU but are cared for on one of the safer, less acute psychiatric units.

Suicide attempts, whether as a result of the distorted thinking of schizophrenia or of profound depression are a common reason for treatment on the psychiatric ICU. Staff follow protocols for meticulous close monitoring so that an untoward, self-destructive event will not be repeated while in care. With a high level of concern, additional precautions are added to safety measures already in place. Bathrooms already have curtains instead of doors so that a ligature like a torn sheet or pajama bottoms cannot be flung over the upper edge and used as a means of hanging.

There are times when a suicide attempt can be averted.

Sara was a twenty-six-year-old woman with the diagnosis of bor-
derline personality disorder who was hospitalized after a serious
attempt to end her life by hanging herself. She was depressed when
she was first admitted but gradually became less so. She was pleas-
ant to all who worked with her and would readily show her rather
dry sense of humor.

Sara, a likable woman, made a sufficient connection with staff
so that they wanted to do whatever they could to help her make
use of her time in the hospital and regain feelings of a good and
stable mood. She expressed interest in learning how to crochet and
a mental health specialist, an accomplished craftsperson, gave her
equipment and instruction. It looked like she was quickly master-
ing the craft but when her teacher wondered why the hat she was
working on didn't appear to be the correct shape, Sara smiled and
said, "It's not a hat. It's a noose." So much for crochet in the ICU.

And sometimes a suicide attempt cannot be deterred…

Lucy, another woman with borderline personality disorder, was
also twenty-six but even more ill than Sara. Ever since early ado-
lescence she had one goal: to kill herself. She would stop eating as
a means to starve herself to death. Nothing could convince her that
life was worth living. Exhausted by multiple attempts to end her life
at home, especially when least expected, her family felt that they
could no longer care for her.

Lucy was now in the ICU after trying to hang herself on a less
restrictive psychiatric unit. She'd had to stay in the medical ICU
then, when sufficiently recovered, it was thought that she'd be safer
with more intense monitoring.

Suicide was always a topic she raised with her staff. At one point, she convinced those who worked with her that she was feeling well and no longer needed an individual monitor with her at all times. She expressed hope that her family would consider taking her home. Routine monitoring continued. A unit monitor makes rounds to check on each patient every fifteen minutes. Lucy precisely timed these rounds. After the monitor noted her quietly resting in her room, she withdrew the strips of sheet she had hidden under her blanket and secured them around her neck. By a fortunate coincidence, another staff member looked in on her since she hadn't appeared for evening snack, found her and called for help, and this patient's life was saved.

An impulsive suicide attempt, completed in moments, may have consequences that can last for a lifetime. Two patients provide examples:

A young man with casts on three limbs and extensive rehabilitation had the diagnosis of schizophrenia. He'd decided that he would rather die if he couldn't escape from his previous hospitalization at another institution where he'd, flung himself from an open third-floor window. After surgery and stabilization in the trauma unit he spent months in the psychiatric ICU and, with the aid of medicine and care, began to regain his will to live.

Just as impulsive was a young psychotic man who decided to die by stretching himself out on the railroad track, believing that spirits living within him instructed him to do this. He didn't die but lost a leg and severely damaged his remaining three limbs. With unremitting delusions that he was governed by forces who had commandeered his body and brain, he remained in the psychiatric ICU while receiving multiple, frequent visits from the orthopedic and rehabilitation services and intensive psychiatric care where his mood improved and his psychosis gradually began to remit.

Violence is always on the mind of everyone who works on the ICU. Unprovoked acts of aggression can come from nowhere while, at other times, staff is aware of which patient has the potential to explode in rage. Training in self-defense moves is helpful but a dangerous patient may need to be contained with the additional aid of security services in order to protect staff and patients from serious injury.

Patient KL, an autistic and schizophrenic man known for violent outbursts, had been in the ICU for months. There was no facility where he could safely live so he remained on the wait list for the state hospital, a list that could remain stagnant for a long time. Although he'd looked calm for the days preceding the event, he unexpectedly entered the nursing station where a nurse was working at a computer. Standing behind her, he placed his hands around her neck in a choke hold. Fortunately, the nurse—a short, slightly built woman—held an expert's belt in martial arts and quickly saved herself from what could have been a disaster. Later, when KL was asked why he tried to choke the nurse, he had no memory of the event. He returned to his calm state and resumed pleasant interactions with staff and even with the nurse he'd unwittingly tried to harm.

This patient could have been charged with assaulting a health care worker, a state crime. Psychiatric staff were reported by the Bureau of Labor Statistics in 2015 to endure workplace violence sixty-nine times greater than the national average. If the physician or staff decide to press charges, the police are called and arrive at the hospital to hear the complaint and speak with the assailant. If taken to jail, the patient may be charged with Third Degree Assault, a Class C felony that carries a potential sentence of one to three months in prison and fines up to $10,000 for a first-time offender. Repeat offenders, may receive a prison term of up to five years.

The attacked person carefully considers whether or not to press charges. Health professionals are trained in a culture of caregiving, so the notion of sending those they have promised to help and protect to jail is distressing. Yet, to endure physical and emotional assault feels defeating for both care provider and patient. Often the decision to prosecute or not is based on whether the patient is too medically compromised or confused to understand what they have done, so police were not called to take KL to jail. His condition prevented him from understanding what he had done, and the conclusion of his care providers was that jail time wouldn't help.

Sometimes there seems no option but to call police and press charges. True, a patient may have mental health issues, but when assault is planned and aimed to kill the care provider, the person is better served in the criminal justice system. There, psychiatric treatment is offered, and providers are protected from violence.

Mary was a street-hardened, heavily tattooed twenty-eight-year-old woman with borderline personality disorder. She had a long history of psychiatric hospitalizations alternating with incarcerations for trespassing, theft, and selling drugs. She would state that she was suicidal, making it impossible to send her home from the Psychiatric Emergency Service, so with threats to run into traffic if discharged, she was admitted to the psychiatric ICU for close monitoring.

After a few days, the treatment team began to make plans for Mary's safety after release from the hospital. Her social worker explored women's shelters as, at the moment, she had no residence to which she could return; appointments were being set with her community psychiatry clinic and insurance issues needed sorting.

One morning, Mary demanded to leave in spite of being told of how many options were being arranged for her well-being. Suddenly, she withdrew a long needle-sharp knife from beneath her sweater and began to scream, "I'm going to kill you," as she lunged after her physician. The physician ran. Staff descended on the assailant, security was called and appeared within moments. It took six men and women to take her to the ground and remove her weapon, a "shiv," a knife fashioned from a hard-plastic dinner tray in a style perfected in prison. Mary was taken off to jail, smiling and joking with the officers who transported her.

Physicians working in the ICU are, like all providers in emergency settings, at high-risk for assault. Even though patient contact may last only for interviewing on rounds, that time can still be tense. The physician is seen as the aggressor, the jailer who forces them to take unwanted medications and keeps them in hospital against their will…so different from staff who change the radio station and supply shampoo and snacks. For safety, physicians must be constantly alert, never seeing a patient alone in their room and always requesting the presence of one or two staff for an interview with an unpredictable and potentially violent person. When endangered, they are encouraged to yell for help from staff while running from immediate danger.

Physicians choose to accept an ICU assignment for individual reasons. Some simply prefer this work to other kinds of psychiatric service. They choose to have short-term connections where they can watch an acutely ill patient stabilize and move on to longer-term care on a less restrictive unit or return to an improved life outside of the hospital. Other doctors spend time working on the ICU because they need to take their obligatory turn as part of their departmental job. Not everyone can have their first-choice assignment, but they have the opportunity to rotate to work in areas that they prefer.

Working in the ICU is challenging but there is a sense of accomplishment at knowing how to stay safe and knowing that the patients treated are being given the best possible chance of stabilization and recovery. The psychiatry ICU runs like an efficient machine. Everyone knows their tasks. All belong to a team with a spirit of watching out for each other, helping the less experienced, and remaining safe. Staff and physicians are proud of the work they do and take satisfaction in seeing their patients improve and be able to move on to the next stage of care.

7

The West Units

With contributions by Heidi Combs, MD and Jay Veitengruber, MD

The two care units located at the opposite end of the hallways from the ICU are 5 West A and 5 West B. They impose fewer restrictions than the ICU, even though these areas remain locked, so hospitalized patients are not free to leave when they choose. Here persons are less ill than those requiring intensive care and more ready to engage in treatment.

In decades past, 5 West A was an unlocked unit. Patients were free to go outside to enjoy the view of Puget Sound or take walks on hospital grounds. They could have outings with visiting family then return to continue care. There were occasions when someone would choose to abandon their hospital treatment and not return, yet these events were surprisingly rare. Currently, with changing times and rules, it has been deemed safer for all if patients remain until they complete treatment. Staff accompany them on outings to a secure courtyard several times a day to try to evade the sometimes-unavoidable sense of confinement.

Before the stricter system was put in place, Serena, a 25-year-old woman with anxiety and depression related to marijuana and cocaine use, was taken off the unit by her visiting case manager to arrange for follow-up appointments off-campus. She excused herself to go to the washroom but didn't return. Several hours later she rang the bell on the door outside of her unit and explained that she was back after getting the fast-food burger she'd been craving for days.

Unlike patients mostly hospitalized in the ICU against their will, there is still a fair number who come to the West Units by their own choice. They may recognize that they are impaired by their serious illness such as schizophrenia, bipolar disorder, personality disorders, depression, or dependency on drugs or alcohol and, for the most part, are ready to accept help. They are admitted as voluntary if they can agree to meet with their team, attend groups, and take medications if prescribed.

Nonetheless, there is a significant number of patients also committed to treatment by state laws. They are able to engage in some treatments and they are in sufficient behavioral control so as not to be violent toward others or try to harm themselves, criteria for an admission or transfer to the ICU.

Diagnoses vary for those on the West Units. Today, moderate depression alone doesn't meet the indication for hospitalization. Individuals qualify for admission if their depression is so severe that they want to end their life, have stopped eating, can no longer care for their own basic needs, or they experience accompanying symptoms of reality-distorting psychosis. A woman with postpartum depression following childbirth may be admitted to prevent her from harming herself or her child as a consequence of her condition. Patients are offered medications, individual and group therapy and, if depression is sufficiently severe, electroconvulsive therapy (ECT) is a helpful and often extremely successful option. Unless ordered by court, the patient can choose whether or not they would like to try ECT as a last resort to attempt to lift intractable depression.

GH is a 65-year-old man who suffered from a depression that severely impaired his thinking. His wife could no longer care for him at home. She placed her husband in a supportive living facility where, because of losing his memory and sense of orientation, he wandered away from his residence and became lost. The police found him sitting on a park bench, disheveled and confused, so GH was taken to the hospital.

His doctor had done everything possible to try to treat this man's condition and, because his impaired thinking, added medications for presumed Alzheimer's dementia. On 5 West B, medicines were continued but, with no improvement seen, ECT seemed a last resort. A usual course of ECT is twelve treatments and, like a curtain lifting from this man's dark life, by treatment number six he began to show interest in going to the dining room for meals. By treatment number ten, he was watching football on TV and recalling the scores. The "pseudo-dementia" that had made him appear cognitively impaired cleared as his depression lifted. Eventually, GH was able to return home and resume his previously enjoyable life.

Patients with psychotic and bipolar disorders are admitted to the West Units. They may be symptomatic, but still able to participate in care. They may be hearing voices but receive no direction to actively harm themselves or someone else. Mania with racing thoughts and rapid speech doesn't prevent treatment.

Patients with dementia are hospitalized on the West Units but never admitted as voluntary because their impaired thinking prevents them from saying that they desire hospitalization. Staff and providers attend to their special medical and emotional needs. Because of their vulnerability, elderly women with dementia are not sent to the Psychiatric ICU because it would be too easy for them to become a victim of violence in this setting.

The scope of diagnostic categories of patients on the West Units is broad. Persons with developmental delay and those on the autism spectrum can be cared for as long as they remain in reasonable behavioral control and show no aggression toward others.

The treatment team—made up of the attending psychiatrist, resident, and medical students—begin rounds on their eight patients at 8 am. The length of time spent with each individual depends on what the patient can tolerate. Some of the more profoundly ill might decline to talk or are able to answer only the most basic questions. They cannot endure sitting to speak with the team, so they are interviewed in their room or in a neutral space. Others can sit with a group and talk for half an hour, giving their history, speaking about events of the previous day, and sharing information about their current state.

The team wants to learn about what is most helpful for the patient. They ask how their attendance in groups is going and what their goals are for the day. They ask if the patient sees benefit in hospitalization. They ask about sleep and appetite and inquire if medications are softening their symptoms or producing side effects. Dosages can be adjusted for maximum positive response and minimum adverse effect. And, of course, every patient is asked about safety and, if they express thoughts of wanting to harm themselves or others, the team requests special, close monitoring by the staff.

After rounds, an interdisciplinary team meeting is held for each of the unit's three teams in order to discuss patient progress and treatment plans. In addition to medical members, present are social workers, nurses, mental health specialists, recreation and occupational therapists, substance use disorder counselors and Peer Specialists—men and woman who have struggled with mental illness themselves and are now well enough to counsel others who are having a similar experience. Meetings occur every weekday. Weekend care is by a covering doctor who attends to patients' immediate needs.

Patients' days are structured to provide maximum therapeutic benefit. Treatment plans are tailored to individual needs and ability to participate. After an initial interview in the morning, members of the medical team return later for longer, in-depth meetings. The pharmacist and social worker may also schedule talks. Throughout the day, various group activities take place and patients are encouraged to attend.

Groups, led by nurses and occupational and recreational therapists, are an important part of care. Exercise classes are organized for different abilities so that even patients with cognitive impairments, physical limitations, or those who have limited concentration can participate and benefit. "Tea group" is quite popular. After performing a tea ceremony, all discuss the reasons they have to feel grateful. Substance use groups are held daily and are attended by those struggling with alcohol and other drugs. 5 West A hosts groups for cognitive behavioral and dialectical behavioral therapies which patients on both units can attend.

Everyone is encouraged to engage in Life Skills group. This activity teaches everyday accomplishments that most take for granted such as going to the grocery store or how to balance a checkbook. Participants discuss how to have successful interactions with others. They learn about having conversations including the topic of when and how to say "no." This is especially important for patients who are vulnerable, struggle with setting personal boundaries, and are prone to be exploited.

Not all patients take medications. Medicines are prescribed to most but, for some, therapy alone is the recommended treatment. For a set of patients with substance use issues, opiate replacement is given to help with cravings and withdrawal but there are others who need to completely detox, get sober, and then learn skills to help maintain sobriety. Meds alone are not the answer.

As on all Harborview's psychiatric units, complicated medical patients are also managed on the less restrictive units. Individuals often have undiagnosed conditions or chronic or acute illnesses that have been ignored while living on the street. Medical attention might have been inadequate or even non-existent, so it is up to the care team to help patients with both their psychiatric and medical troubles. Basic laboratory studies screen for illness and, when suspicions are raised that a complex condition exists, providers request further, more sophisticated tests. Physicians often find untreated hypertension, diabetes, hepatitis, HIV, and urinary tract infections so regimens of care are started that, if followed, will prolong lives. Providers need never feel alone with the problems they confront: The Medical Consult Service is available to offer advice and support.

Patients with longstanding medical and emotional issues can receive treatment that results in a new lease on life.

Jorge, a 31-year-old man with diabetes, was an undocumented immigrant who only spoke Spanish, his native language. Living in a tiny apartment with his mother and very young sisters and brothers, he had to remain in the bedroom as his mother was concerned that the other children would be infected with his diabetes if he socialized or even shared meals with them.

The rules that Jorge had to abide by were even more demor-
alizing. He had to turn out the light in the room at an early hour
and must stay alone in the dark. With his history of sexual abuse
as a child, it is no wonder that this gentle, quiet man, interviewed
through an interpreter, was so overwhelmed by stress that he became
depressed, anxious, and wanted to end his life.

When Jorge first entered 5 West B he was withdrawn and spoke
little to anyone, even avoiding conversation with his Spanish inter-
preter. He was encouraged to attend a cognitive behavioral therapy
group and, so he could participate, was given an instructional book
in Spanish.

Soon after he began attending group, the treatment team noticed
a definite change for the better. He looked brighter, said how much
he was enjoying his group, and felt that he was being helped by what
he learned and felt while attending. In rounds on the following days,
he asked if there were any options for where he might live, knowing
that this would be a challenge for someone unofficially in the US.

Jorge suffered from social anxiety disorder, a condition where
the afflicted person has intense fear of being judged and viewed as
being inadequate. Jorge had these symptoms since he was a teen
when he was thought to be simply shy and not recognized as hav-
ing an illness made worse by the painful living situation he had
to endure. With his diagnosis now recognized and his treatment
begun, Jorge had a new lease on life and no longer wanted it to end.

Safety measures are in place on all inpatient units. Bathroom
doors are replaced with sliding curtains, staff frequently checks
patient rooms, and there is heightened awareness that, without
vigilance, tragedy could occur. If needed, suicide precautions
entail providing the patient with paper rather than cloth garments.
Sheets, pillowcases, and soft blankets that could be torn in strips to

make a ligature are removed from the bed. A staff monitor watches a potentially suicidal patient at all times.

Although observation is meticulous, staff still finds those intent on harming themselves. Personality-disordered patients will fashion a sharp object with which they will cut themselves as a means of expressing their inner pain. They might find something to tie around their neck in a suicide gesture, either serious or just meant for others to see how distressed they are feeling. They may stockpile pills with a plan to overdose. Others, yearning for the drugs they used outside the hospital, will find creative ways to have illicit substances provided by visitors. Administrators regularly assess the units to do everything possible to limit opportunities for self-harm.

Even severely dysregulated patients can be successful treated.

Judy was first admitted to 5 West A at age 21 with a history of over 100 past hospital admissions, some of which were for suicide attempts. Her arms and legs were covered with scars from self-inflicted cuts and burns. Special funding was obtained from the county to try to break this cycle of self-destructive behaviors alternating with hospitalizations that she saw as punitive.

A program was created for Judy to reinforce healthy behaviors. She was scheduled for planned admissions to 5 West A, an event she liked and found helpful, that would happen only if she was attending her individual therapy appointments and had no intervening emergency department visits or other hospitalizations. The treatment plan worked. Although there have been setbacks, three years later she is mostly out of the hospital, lives on her own, and volunteers to help at an animal shelter.

The outcome of another patient who had prolonged stays on the medical and psychiatric units was also considered a success.

Barbara Jean was a 37-year-old woman with diagnoses that remained a puzzle: possible developmental delay complicated by elements of borderline personality disorder. Her continuing and unremitting weight gain to as much as five hundred pounds couldn't be halted. She would take food from others and call for pizza delivery. She had wounds on her abdomen and legs that never healed as she persisted in disrupting them, perhaps as a passive and distorted attempt at suicide. This behavior resulted in bouts of sepsis, necessitating stays in the medical intensive care unit.

This unfortunate woman who had no friends, family, or outside life, remained at Harborview for years. After many trials, a successful behavioral plan was finally devised. She liked 5 West A as she felt comfortable with the staff and her limited activities. If she acted out by attempting to harm others or disrupted her wounds, she would have to transfer to a more restrictive unit until she could regain self-control. After some months of this program, she was finally ready to leave the hospital and was accepted at an adult family home outside of Seattle. Like many others, she left the hospital with a smile but adamantly swore that she would never need to return.

Discharge planning can pose challenges. There are times when a personality-disordered patient will profess to be suicidal. They will threaten to end their life unless provided with housing, an option that cannot realistically be fulfilled by social work following release from inpatient status.

Many questions need answers and social work and the medical team combine efforts to arrange the safest and best discharge plan. There are often few options. Will the patient go to a shelter, to their home, or to stay with family? Will they remain in Washington or need assistance to travel to another state? Where will they receive psychiatric care and, if they have accompanying physical conditions, medical treatment? All plans need to be set so that the patient stands the best chance of things going well after the hospital stay. The relationship with the inpatient psychiatrist and team ends with discharge. Patients will now work with doctors, nurse practitioners, and therapists who continue care in a community mental health center or office outpatient setting.

In spite of the many issues that arise in caring for the severely mentally ill, the hundreds of patients treated each year on the forty-five beds on 5 West A and B have a better future as a result of their hospital stay.

8

Social Work on the Inpatient Units

With contributions by Barbara Kleweno, MSW;
Molly McNamara, MSW, LICSW; and Cord Pryse, MSW, LICSW

The importance of the treatment team's social workers cannot be over-emphasized. They meet their patient on arrival to their unit and work with them throughout their hospital stay. Patients are generally much more kindly disposed toward their social worker than the medical members of their team, as this clinician doesn't tell them that they cannot have their freedom and leave, nor does the social worker make them take medicine or insist that they shower and keep their room tidy. The social worker is someone on their side with plenty of help on offer.

Each inpatient unit has a social worker with a caseload of ten or eleven patients. They gather information about the patient's history and supports that can be relied on after hospitalization. There may be a mental health case manager with whom the social worker will connect in order to best coordinate post-hospital care. The patient might have been living at a facility such as an adult family or nursing home and it will be the social worker who explores if a return is feasible. The social worker clarifies funding, financial resources, and insurance status. In short, their goal is to help the patient, when stable, return to his community as safely as possible.

Coordination of care after an unexpected discharge can be challenging. If the judge decides that there are insufficient grounds for hospital detainment, it's the social worker's task to hurriedly create a workable plan that includes a place to stay and a way to get there and, if the patient wishes, an appointment for mental health follow-up. With an unexpected discharge, the luxury of having sufficient time to prepare just isn't there.

Most often patients demand to leave the hospital no matter the state of their mental or physical health. Occasionally, the social worker must face a patient who refuses discharge. "I'm not leaving until I get housing" is a declaration all-too-frequently heard. Unfortunately, permanent housing is very, very scarce in Seattle and finding an apartment—if one can be found at all—can be a project that extends over years. The inpatient social worker can only initiate the process by referral to the case manager who works with the community agency to place the patient on the long housing wait list.

Charles, a 39-year-old homeless man, had an extensive history of psychiatric hospital admissions for feeling either suicidal or homicidal and emergency department visits mostly for intoxication with alcohol or illegal substances. His times between hospital stays were punctuated by sojourns at various jails and, for one three-year period, incarceration in the penitentiary for attacking a "friend" with a switchblade knife, a crime he denied having committed.

Charles was admitted through Harborview's Psychiatric Emergency Service with the complaint of feeling suicidal and having a plan to jump from the Aurora Bridge, Seattle's highest. Although his past included actual acts of self-harm by cutting on his arms and running into oncoming traffic, he was often under the influence of alcohol or other drugs when these occurred.

During his current admission that coincided with the gray, chilly Seattle late fall, he spent most of his time in his room listening to the radio. If he didn't receive a snack or shoes from the donation closet as soon as he asked for them, he would throw an object or punch the staff who didn't immediately respond to his request. This went on for several days and it became apparent that he was neither participating in treatment nor having symptoms for which medications would benefit. He was vague about ongoing feelings of wanting to kill himself but insisted on remaining in the hospital until he could get an apartment despite that he was informed that this involved a very long process and couldn't be accomplished as an inpatient. He seemed ready for discharge but refused referral to a shelter nor would he consider a stay at Crisis Respite Service.

Social work paid numerous visits to Charles both as part of routine care and as a response to his urgent requests. Finally, the entire team concurred that Charles wasn't benefitting from a longer hospital stay and that it was time for discharge. After months of contacting various placement possibilities, the persistent social worker found unexpected success: An adult family home said, "Welcome Charles!" With a prescription for an anti-depressant in hand and a broad grin on his face, he was discharged to his new home, pleased that people were willing to give him a chance.

Housing options are scarce, but social workers try their best to find a match for their patient. If the person has Medicaid and is connected to a community mental health program, additional resources, although with limited availability, can be found through their agency. If a patient has chronic mental illness, they need more support than a shelter could offer. King County has a residential program that is, sadly, usually full and unable to accommodate new applicants. Other facilities called "group homes," geared to residents with mental health needs, offer three levels of care: standard supportive housing, supervised living, and long-term care. These, too, are often out of reach because of their long wait list.

Another option, also available only after a wait of weeks to months, is the adult family home (AFH). To access this option, the Home and Community Services agency becomes involved. An AFH is a residential home licensed to care for up to six non-related clients. They provide room, board, laundry, necessary supervision, and, if needed, help with personal care, and social services. Placement, as will many other residential options, is dependent on the amount of money the patient's insurance will pay.

Unlike involuntary hospitalization, these facilities are unlocked, and residents may leave if they choose. If, on the other hand, the person becomes violent, the caregiver can call the police for removal back to the hospital.

The social worker may take the patient to visit the care facility to see if it would be a good fit for both. Before travel, the safety of this outing is assessed as carefully as possible but even with the best of intentions, untoward events can occur.

One social worker who usually has no problems escorting patients to visit potential housing options, recalls several harrowing experiences. A patient bolted out of the car while still in the hospital parking lot. Rather than risk injury, she let the patient go and was prepared to notify police if he didn't return...which he did with a cigarette in hand after several tense minutes went by.

The same social worker was driving across the bridge over Puget Sound when the patient angrily demanded to be let out of the car while pushing the unlock button and maintaining a steady stare. Before they arrived at the facility, the patient had calmed sufficiently so that a burger at McDonald's was enough to make for a successful and safe visit.

The most challenging placements are for those with dementia or developmental delay. Individuals with intellectual disability are managed by the Developmental Disabilities Administration (DDA), an agency of Washington's Department of Health and Human Services. This agency monitors the well-being of approximately 50,000 child and adult clients. Although they are undeniably conscientious, they still must contend with the paucity of residential placements. When one cannot be readily found and the person is still legally detained in the hospital, then they are placed on the wait list for the DDA unit at Western State Hospital, another setting where openings are only rarely available.

Bobby was a 29-year-old man from Arkansas who had never actually been registered with his state's DDA. His elderly guardian in his home state could no longer care for him so, with the best of intentions, bought Bobby a plane ticket to Seattle where he could live with a cousin. Bobby wandered away from the cousin's house and, when picked up by police, refused to return. The kindly officers kept him at the police station, unwilling to send him back to the street and, not knowing what else to do, finally took him to Harborview.

Bobby hated his time in the hospital, repeatedly demanding then begging to leave, screaming that he preferred being on the street to being at Harborview. Sending him out on his own with no supportive services was not an option. Complicating the situation was that Washington's DDA cannot assume responsibility for an out-of-state unregistered person.

Because he unable to control his impulse to hit others, he had to remain on the Psychiatric Intensive Care Unit where dangerous behaviors can be more closely monitored than in less restrictive settings. As he entered a period of calm, his social worker was able to find an adult family home willing to accept him.

The staff celebrated his achievement with a pizza party and sent him on his way to his new home.

Finding a place to live for someone with dementia poses an equal challenge. There is no agency comparable to the DDA for the cognitively compromised elderly.

Social work was confronted with a particularly difficult case. A woman who appeared to be in her early 60s came to the Psychiatric Emergency Service and requested hospital admission. She had been living on the street and didn't know her name or where she had come from.

Social work's detective skills were called into action. After months in the hospital, the patient, referred to as "Jane Doe," finally remembered her first name then her surname. She incidentally mentioned the name of a small Seattle business. When that company was contacted, the current owner recalled that his partner, long deceased, had told him of a daughter who disappeared. As the pieces fell into place, the Harborview patient was identified as the missing daughter who was an heiress with a sizeable fortune. With the aid of a newly appointed guardian, this woman now had an identity and could be placed safely in secure housing for those suffering with dementia. A good solution to a perplexing puzzle.

This is just one example of the many skills that social work calls into action every day!

9

The Medical Student Experience

By Ari Azani, BA; Stephen R. Durkee, BA;
Jocelyn C. McCornack, BS; and Amanda Sekijima, BS
With a contribution by Paul Borghesani, MD, PhD, Director,
Psychiatry Clerkship University of Washington School of Medicine

After two years of instruction in the science of medicine, students are now introduced to clinical work. In their six weeks' psychiatry clerkship they gain a foundation that will prove useful for their entire medical career. Here they learn to talk to patients about topics that are difficult to raise like suicide, psychosis and what goes on in the minds of the mentally ill. It's not easy to ask if someone is feeling like ending their life or to hear about delusions that plague their waking hours. But under the guidance and supervision of residents and attending physicians, trainees are encouraged to feel at ease when asking hard questions whose answers are necessary for competent and compassionate care.

Students learn that psychiatry is more than making a diagnosis and prescribing a medication. Memorizing the DSM-5, the specialty's diagnostic bible, and understanding every word in a psychopharmacology textbook is not all to mastering psychiatry. Although learning the basics of illness identification, investigation and treatment is necessary, spending time with their patients is the vital element of student education and an important focus of the rotation.

Students are encouraged to have conversations in as normal a manner as possible and ask about patients' lives. What was it like growing up? What was your family like? How about school? Who are the special people in your life now? What are your feelings about psychiatry and medical doctors? What would you like to see happen in your future? Building rapport is the ultimate and often challenging goal.

Student Ari Azani shares his experience:

While I did not have experience working with patients with mental illness, my interest and enthusiasm as a medical student, rather than my expertise, made me feel like an asset to the team. I learned that by just sitting and listening to my patients each afternoon, I would have the opportunity to shed light on the lives of those who were reluctant to speak during morning rounds.

During the second week of my rotation, a depressed middle-aged woman with bipolar disorder agreed, with family encouragement, to hospitalization. She was withdrawn and wouldn't look at us. She stared at the ground and spoke so softly as to be almost inaudible. When asked why she was at Harborview, she looked vacant and didn't reply. Each morning, she would sit to join us in the interview room for rounds then immediately stand up to leave. Each afternoon I would talk to her and try to learn more about her life. She remained guarded and refused to tell us anything about herself. Upon noticing that she ate little at meals, I encouraged her to talk about her dietary restrictions with staff. One day, without warning, she began to speak about her love of dancing and how she missed going to dance class. As we built rapport, she began accepting treatment by attending groups and taking medicine which she had previously refused. Her goal changed from wanting to leave, to wanting to go home and dance again.

Each patient is unique, and it is their life situation, not simply their diagnosis, which dictates the plan. For my patient, adherence to medication is important, but the intention to return to the dance floor is essential as well. I chose psychiatry to find the right piece of the puzzle of my patient's life, that will help them feel whole again.

Students are a working part of the treatment team comprised of a resident, attending physician and possibly a fellow student as well as the social worker and nursing staff. The morning begins with the team meeting where staff report overnight events. Response to medicines are noted and, if needed, alterations in dose or type are made. The team is alert to changes in behavior. Everyone looks at what has helped make improvements in thinking and attitude. Finally, the social worker explores housing options to follow discharge as the patient nears the end of their hospital stay.

At the end of morning meeting, rounds begin. Physicians and students invite the patient to a room where all may sit for the interview. If too ill or dysregulated to tolerate joining the team, the interview can be conducted at the bedside or in another more comfortable location. The student leads the interview of their own patient with the team ready to ask questions and offer support.

There are times when a patient is uncomfortable with having to reveal intimate information to a large group. Understanding this reluctance, the student will invite the patient to speak in a more private setting with just the two of them present. There are other times when the patient says that they refuse to talk about themselves with someone who is "merely" a student and will only agree to meet with the attending physician. Patient preferences are respected. Often, such an individual might have some peripheral interaction with the student and, finding that person an attentive and caring listener, will go on to have a satisfying relationship with the trainee they previously rejected on the basis of inexperience.

After rounds, students and physicians gather to review what they have learned about all of the team's patients. Trainees hear a critique of their interview and get suggestions for future changes. This meeting then shifts into an educational mode. Attendings may teach about a topic relevant to a patient whose condition is current or discuss a subject of common concern such as antipsychotic medication, psychosis or chemical dependency.

Student Jocelyn McCornack remember the start of her rotation:

I can recall my first day on the ward, observing my attending with our patients. I remember paying careful attention to every bit of body language, both hers and the patients. I remember each measure she took to ensure her own and the patient's safety, like standing at the doorway in such a way that no one felt boxed in. She would speak in a firm, direct, but very calm tone. She was always nonplussed if the patient was too upset to speak and would calmly end the interview if the patient couldn't answer questions. It made it much easier for me to begin my first interview, which happened soon afterwards.

After a few days, I was assigned my own patient. I began by introducing myself and asked about his mood, his sleep and his appetite, but his abrupt answers became loud and pressured, and he grew visibly upset and started to shout. I did my best to counteract his escalating energy with an especially calm tone, but it became apparent he couldn't continue. We quickly concluded the interview and I consoled myself with the thought that improvement was a process that doesn't occur overnight. Over two weeks he responded to medicines and to the calming atmosphere of the Intensive Care Unit. Eventually he was able to answer my questions and we could discuss what was happening to him now and what he'd like his future to be.

Despite all of my initial apprehension, I grew comfortable with talking about suicide and asking about thoughts of violence and harming others. I aimed to create an atmosphere in which the patient could feel comfortable, as well.

In the afternoon, students address tasks necessary for good care. With their patient's permission, they call relatives and friends to learn what their life was like before hospitalization. With or without permission, as permitted by law, the trainee calls current or previous providers to gather clinical information. If safe and appropriate, the student then returns to spend time with their patient. This is the opportunity to build confidence in interviewing skills and to form their own style of approach. These special moments contribute to some of the most meaningful times of the rotation. Working with the same patient each day provides continuity for student and patient alike.

Student Amanda Sekijima recalls:

The same year I entered college, my little sister was diagnosed with schizophrenia. Our normal lives disappeared, and her condition strained our family. Given my personal experience with mental illness, I started my psychiatry rotation scared yet curious and eager. I felt I had unique insight into mental illness, but would this translate into better or worse care for patients? I was unsure how I would respond to psychiatric patients, especially if their narrative happened to be similar to my sister's story. I voiced my concerns with my attendings and from the beginning they offered support and reassurance, so I never felt alone.

My fear of my sister's narrative being comparable to those I heard at work was confirmed. Yet, my personal experiences didn't make interactions more difficult to navigate, but rather equipped me with compassion. Considering my family history, I felt I could better understand my patients' perspective of illness.

I think that nothing in medicine or society is more stigmatized than mental illness. My experience caring for certain patients reinforced my plan to become a psychiatrist. I wanted to help them and learn how to do this in the best way possible. I realized that developing a therapeutic alliance with a patient is a dynamic and sometimes irregular process that requires effort. I experienced awkward moments when I felt clumsy and I couldn't adequately articulate my thoughts, and so the therapeutic relationship suffered. I would turn to my supervisors and talk about what had been happening. They helped me find different and more effective strategies, advice I gratefully appreciated.

Mrs. B, a seventy-year-old woman was depressed and profoundly hopeless. She catastrophized everything, including what would or would not be served at dinner. She believed that every treatment would fail. It was emotionally exhausting for me to provide the same reassurances each day that all seemed to go nowhere. Eventually, she got better with ECT and, as her depression lifted, our therapeutic alliance improved.

I came to realize that fostering a healthy treatment relationship requires constant maintenance, and just like any other relationship there is room for error and clarification.

My experiences taught me to have the courage to relate to patients much different from myself.

Formal weekly teaching sessions are offered for all students on the rotation. These didactics, presented by attending psychiatrists and senior residents, offer basic topics in psychiatry. Presentations are designed to be interactive; teachers and trainees discuss cases to illustrate the subject at hand. Students are encouraged to ask questions and contribute material from their own experience.

Dr. Paul Borghesani, Director of the Psychiatry Clerkship, explains to students:

You aren't required to know everything, but you are required to know as much as you can about your patient and their problems. So, I don't want to inundate you with a lot of formal lectures that would force you to do tons of outside study. I'd rather give you time to learn as much as you can about patients and their needs. And I hope that's true across all disciplines. The goal of didactics is to provide education because I think it's good to have it, but it's not meant to be 'this is our syllabus, and this is what's really essential to you.' It's more like 'here are some lectures and we hope you can learn from them. These are things to think about and they will be your building blocks for future study.' The challenge of being a doctor is that you're always learning.

Of the twenty or so students on their psychiatry rotation, one third is assigned to the psychiatric intensive care unit and the others are divided between the two less restrictive settings. All are instructed in safety behaviors. At the mid-point of their six-week rotation, they change teams so that all can experience the variety of illnesses treated on the different units. Patients on all units represent individuals with more severe mental illness than seen in other facilities around the northwest region.

Education covers many aspects of care. During their six weeks at Harborview, students take shifts in the Psychiatric Emergency Service to see people as they enter the system for evaluation. This is the time before patients get medicines to help calm agitation, when they might still be under the influence of mind-altering substances or when they are acute in their desire to harm themselves or others. During the rotation students are invited to witness administration of electroconvulsive therapy, an effective treatment for depression and other intractable conditions. Harborview is one of the few facilities in the region to offer this modality. Contrary to what some students would like, the rotation doesn't afford an outpatient experience as patients would be reluctant to have an observer present for an appointment that is designed to be a private meeting with their provider.

Student Stephen Durkee shares his experience:

GH was a twenty-year-old woman who presented as acutely psychotic to the emergency department. Her urine analysis showed that she had methamphetamines in her system. From the size of her abdomen, she appeared somewhere in her third trimester of pregnancy. I'd just finished my OB/GYN rotation and was particularly aware of what expectant mothers could be going through.

Gradually, I pieced together GH's story. She'd had a hard time at school and left before finishing. Her life afterwards was dominated by drugs and sex trafficking. She'd had one supportive relationship that ended when her boyfriend, the father of her child, was killed in a car accident. She had only rare contact with her family who weren't likely to help her and the new baby. To make matters even worse, the current man in her life was leading her down a path of destruction.

Shortly after admission, GH wanted to be discharged. None of the legitimate causes that would prolong her hospital stay were present, so we had to let her go. The day she was released, I was pondering the four principles of ethics I learned in medical school: autonomy, nonmaleficence, beneficence and justice. I wasn't sure we were precisely abiding by all of these, but the chief principle we operated under that day was autonomy. She had the right to return to her own life, even if it ultimately harmed her.

I wanted to help GH by arranging a better life for her. Of course, this couldn't happen. Though my vision for GH was naïve and probably idealistic, I want to always nourish and maintain this kind of compassion.

Despite the missing element of participating in outpatient clinics, the rotation offers a comprehensive view of psychiatric care. Rather than as a means to sell a psychiatric career to students, faculty has designed the experience with the goal of educating trainees about mental illness and to foster comfort with speaking with those who are ill, a skill that will serve them well for the rest of their medical career.

Nursing: The Heart of Inpatient Care

With contributions by Elizabeth Bofferding, RN, BSN;
Barbara L. Fowler, RN, BSN; Susan Johnson, RN; Wyeth
Johnston, RN; and Chris Sheets, DNP, RN

Staff hold the front line for inpatient care. Working on the psychiatric ICU are nurses, mental health specialists and hospital assistants who take vital signs, check each patient on walk-around rounds, and sit with a person needing individual monitoring. For an entire shift that can last for as many as twelve hours, staff work with only timed breaks for meals and rest. Because of high acuity and need, there's a low patient-to-employee ratio so each person gets concentrated care and attention for the entire shift.

Patient management is challenging. Staff must work with people who don't necessarily want care or may be unable to realize that they need it. Patients often don't recognize that their illness is preventing them from being out in the world. They are unaware that life could be better, and that inpatient treatment is the first step to success outside of the hospital.

At times, staff face a moral predicament because knowing what is best for the patient doesn't always feel right at the time. For example, the nurse knows that antipsychotic medication is necessary because disorganization and delusions are unlikely to go away without it, yet the individual may resist as they don't understand the need. The nurse prefers to be able to convince the person to accept medicine but, if unsuccessful, state law permits giving an injection against the patient's will. In such an instance and in spite of training in safe procedures, staff still remains at risk for harm when medicine must be forced.

An additional challenge is needing to watch for the onset of acute medical conditions. Knowing when to respond to physical signs or to a complaint, no matter how vaguely expressed, can be a life or death matter. In their state of mental turmoil, a patient may be unable to clearly describe their physical distress; it is staff's responsibility to be constantly on alert.

Even though all nurses have received extensive training, those who come to work on a psychiatric unit may lack sufficient practical experience to attend to patients with medical needs. To address this issue and to help the nurse gain competence, staff is aided by support and instruction from Harborview's clinical educators and wound care specialists.

Harborview's nurse educators provide guidance in how to perform procedures such as inserting a feeding tube when a psychiatric patient refuses to eat or in monitoring for certain disease signs. Educators offer formally organized training opportunities for Harborview nurses in other specialties as well as for those in the community.

Nurses look after their patients' wounds, often sustained from living on the street and being prone to receiving blows, burns, and cuts. A person might have a wound that needs attention after having been transferred from a medical or surgical service for continued psychiatric care. With evaluation, instruction, and support from Harborview's wound care team staffed by nurses certified in their specialty, psychiatric nurses may give treatments and change dressings.

Experiences on each shift vary and are often unpredictable. If their patient is calm, cooperative and appreciative of care, that's fine. But, so often, this is not the case, especially with those held in the Intensive Care Unit against their will. Staff must contend with agitation and aggression. Patients may want to harm others and make staff a target. Violence can erupt without warning and, when this occurs, multiple employees converge to keep the individual from harming themselves and those around them. Although staff have been trained in safety techniques, takedowns during an agitated outburst still pose significant risk.

When patients are considered particularly dangerous, they are secluded in their rooms or, if unable to remain in control, they are physically restrained for safety, a procedure considered a last resort. To safely render care or provide food and hygiene, staff enter the room with one or more partners. If credible threats are made, safety officers accompany the team. The very number of those present including uniformed men and women is usually enough to deter even the most violent aggressor.

Over the years, nurses and their associates have sustained significant injuries. An older mental health specialist was the repeated target of a psychotic and antisocial patient who wanted to damage his eyes. After several attempts and in spite of the worker's vigilance, the patient did inflict an injury serious enough to require surgery and weeks away from work for recovery.

Both male and female staff have been pushed, punched, bitten, scratched, tripped, and hit causing injuries. One nurse's kidneys were damaged after being punched. That same nurse sustained a herniated disc in a fall during a takedown. Some injuries have been significant, resulting in staff retirement or the decision to leave their job. Other injuries result in less physical damage, but high emotional impact. After an assault, staff gather in the nursing station to talk about what happened, discuss what might have been done differently to try to avoid a repeat of the event, and to generally support each other through a stressful and traumatic event.

Even if there's no violence, nurses must contend with angry patients who scream, call names, and refuse medicine. Nurse Barbara Fowler explains:

> In situations like that, I just try to be an active listener. I aim to validate what they're saying. A lot of times, these people are so used to not being heard and not having their feelings affirmed that screaming and name-calling is the only response they know. But you can crack through their shell of rage by actually sitting down and asking what's going on. I let them know that I'm here to help. Sometimes that will melt their anger and sometimes not. I know that names don't hurt so I just keep going and hope that I will eventually make a breakthrough. I just be as professional as I can be, and there are times when it's easier than others.

There is always a shortage of nurses willing to work on the psychiatric intensive care unit because of the demands and risks associate with the job. Younger nurses stay for a few years then perhaps join a program to get an advanced degree or just feel that they no longer want to work in such an intense environment and move on to other positions. Yet some older staff have continued at their post for decades. They are ready to accept risk; they are comfortable with their skills, truly love their work, and are proud to make their contribution caring for this under-served population.

Nurses have a full day, evening, or night of work. They are tasked with reviewing all patient orders placed by the medical teams. They monitor patients' food intake; inadequate nutrition can result from psychosis or depression. Because excessive weight gain has been a problem on account of medications, boredom, and inactivity, nurses have spearheaded the transition from giving puddings and ice cream as snacks to having fruit, yogurt, and sugar-free Jell-O on offer. Patients haven't seemed to mind this shift and these healthier options are consistent with good hospital care.

Chris Sheets, RN, recalls the challenges of working with a group of patients in the ICU:

Because there's no place else for them to go, Harborview cares for a population of autistic and developmentally disabled patients. Sometimes they can stay with us for a year or even longer because no one can find a safe placement for them.

I recall one patient in particular. He was a young man with fetal alcohol syndrome and a very low IQ. He wanted to leave the hospital but was totally unable to make a plan for self-care. He wouldn't know how to access a shelter or get food. Unbelievably, the court let him go when his case for commitment was heard. He was excited to get out of doors but then when he realized he had no place to go, he was afraid to leave.

I, too, was scared for him. Thankfully, we were able to find a place in Harborview's new shelter where he stayed overnight then, in the morning, we were able to encourage him to return to the hospital. I'd worried about him the whole night.

Another nurse recalls patient Freddie, a thirty-five-year-old man with severe autism:

Freddie came to us from a local hospital that just couldn't manage him. He'd run around and swing at people, sometimes hitting them and sometimes barely missing. He wasn't able to speak. Some of the nurses had become really attached to him and were quite sad when he finally left to go to Western State Hospital. I always cared for him when it was my assignment, but I just never felt a connection to him. We're all different.

Nurse Sheets remembers cases that had successful outcomes:

We care for patients on our unit who've had successful lives before they became ill. Lawyers, teachers, college students, and even a medical student. They come to us because they're too ill to be hospitalized on a less restrictive unit or even at another hospital.

A nurse practitioner student had had several manic breaks by the time she arrived here. As ill as she was, she hated her condition and really wanted to get well. She worked hard at taking her medicines and, although not always successful, tried to cooperate with the staff. Eventually, she was sufficiently recompensated for transfer to one of our less-restrictive units and finally was ready for discharge. I was so pleased to learn that she returned to school and was stable and well in the community.

Nurse Sheets adds:

It's hard to see someone from your own profession who is so ill but it's great to see them getting better.

He goes on to say:

Psychiatry is a good place to learn about yourself. Above all, we discover patience. We've all had our life struggles and here we learn about the challenges that others face. We try to understand what they're going through but, if we can't, it doesn't matter. We just need to be there and give them our support.

One senior nurse identifies the need to understand himself to achieve a greater appreciation of the patient's situation, recognizing that the years behind give him the advantage over younger and less seasoned nurses.

When I explain something to a patient, I can sometimes say, "I wish someone had had that conversation with me twenty years ago." I want to help a patient see that they have a future. My empathy for their situation is greater today because of my past life experience.

Whether nurses have worked on the ICU for three years or three decades, their commitment to service is unshakable.

Elizabeth Bofferding, RN, came to Harborview from a background of working in facilities serving those with dementia and autism. She identified the similarities in behaviors in the psychotic, manic, and illegal drug-influenced patients on the ICU and was prepared to tolerate unpleasant behaviors.

We see patients at their worst, and we get the chance to make them feel like they matter and have our support. That may be a new experience for them. I like watching people get better. I take pride in working with the most challenging patients in the region and I like working on a team that really cares about these people who are often ignored by the rest of the world.

Over the past few years, our patients seem to have more and more complicated medical conditions. And when illness is bad, their mind is affected. You see a person's mental state deteriorate as their physical health declines.

Sometimes we have to be happy with small victories. I had a patient who was a severe diabetic. I had to tell him, "You can't have a peanut butter sandwich with extra jelly. Your blood sugar was sky high this morning." It was a triumph when he agreed to eat an apple for a snack. Finally allowing us to check his sugars three times a day was an even greater accomplishment.

Because of the difficulty of finding a suitable placement, patients can remain in the hospital for a long time. Staff may become invested in the care of a particular patient they have worked with for weeks and even months. They form a relationship based on developing trust, a condition from which all involved benefit.

Although each nurse works with their patient in their own individual style, they still set a general care plan to be followed by all. A uniform approach, identifying necessary boundaries and conveying a sense of consistency, is vital to good care.

A full complement of nurses also works on the West Units where the patients are less acutely ill than those on the ICU. Those patients usually have both psychiatric and addiction issues. The unit 5 West A has a focus of treating the problems caused by personality disorders. Although actively suicidal patients are generally admitted to the ICU, the unit 5 West B will still take them on, providing a constant observer to ensure their safety.

A nurse describes events that have occurred:

We had one patient who tried to hang himself and another who mutilated himself with scissors. We had been watching them closely but when a person is absolutely determined to harm themselves, it is almost impossible to prevent it. They might suddenly have begun to respond to the voices they're hearing so their actions can be unexpected and unpredictable.

Similar to nursing tasks on the ICU, West Unit nurses pass medications, attend family meetings to discuss progress and plans, help with serving meals, and do safety checks of rooms to make sure no hazardous or contraband materials are present. They are available to support their patients when the need for comfort and explanations arise and to intervene if they notice developing anger or aggression. They are also trained to lead therapeutic groups such as those providing cognitive behavioral therapy for depression and dialectical behavioral therapy to address the problems and behavioral dysregulation of borderline personality disorder.

Nurses on the West Units, like ICU nurses, feel a sense of responsibility and commitment to the patients cared for over time. Often, patients return for repeat hospitalizations. When learning about the death of a man who had been admitted many times on the various psychiatric units, Nurse Susan Johnson sums up the feelings of many:

It hit us hard. Over the years that we cared for J, we saw him at his worst and we always thought that there was some hope when he was discharged. But he'd always come back to us, sometimes in worse condition than ever. He used methamphetamine and he used to repeatedly harm himself. But we were always glad to be able to take care of him. When it came down to it, Harborview was all he had, and the nurses were proud to be a bright spot in his life—even if it wasn't for long.

11

Pharmacy for Psychiatry

With contributions by Chelsea Markle, PharmD,
BCPP and Jennifer Jepson, PharmD, BCPS

Pharmacists are indispensable for patient care. As specialists trained in prescribing psychiatric medications, they advise the treatment team in managing psychosis, violence, mania, and the myriad problems patients demonstrate. Pharmacists attend morning and afternoon reports where staff and providers set the day's treatment plan. They are on call to visit with a person reluctant to take their medicines; they sit with the patient to explain why treatment is needed and gently describe expected results as well as possible side effects. Pharmacists are available to the team by phone for immediate consultation. In addition to patient care, they offer a weekly meeting for physicians and medical students to provide education and support. In short, the psychiatric services couldn't operate without the aid of the pharmacist.

Two pharmacists serve Harborview's 66-bed inpatient units. Both advise providers in the outpatient setting as well. In these areas they implement educational opportunities to keep everyone informed about current advances in psychopharmacology.

Chelsea Markle has been the consultant pharmacist for psychiatry since 2005. After obtaining her Doctor of Pharmacy degree, she completed a general pharmacy practice residency and became board certified in psychiatric pharmacy. She was drawn to work with the underserved, so Harborview was the ideal match. Jennifer Jepsen is the second inpatient pharmacist who's certified in pharmacotherapy and maintains a similar devotion to her patients and hospital.

At Harborview pharmacists can help people with schizophrenia and bipolar disorder who are homeless and ill, sometimes with a multitude of accompanying medical diseases. Many are admitted because they stopped taking their medicine, so the pharmacist looks at the barriers that have gotten in the way of compliance. Each conversation is different, depending on how much the patient can understand. This is an art they've developed over time to tailor discussions to what an individual can tolerate and absorb.

The pharmacists' goal is to encourage acceptance of needed medication. Having to keep track of too many pills can be overwhelming, so the pharmacist refines post-discharge regimens to keep the number of prescribed drugs to the minimum. On the less-restrictive units, with the assistance of occupational therapy, the pharmacist leads groups to teach the importance of recognizing the need for medicines and to identify ways of making it easier to take them.

The pharmacist doesn't prescribe medications but works with the treatment team to best select medicines that will be most effective in the shortest amount of time. To do the job with accuracy, the pharmacist must be familiar with the latest research so she can recommend the most evidence-based treatments.

Schizophrenia, a common illness affecting about one percent of the population, is a condition where connection with reality is lost. It is difficult to treat, as some "positive" symptoms like hallucinations, delusions of paranoia, and having disorganized thoughts ultimately may only be reduced rather than eliminated. The "negative" symptoms of schizophrenia are even more resistant to treatment. These manifestations cause patients to withdraw and lose any joy of living they experienced before becoming ill.

Patients are prescribed antipsychotics, medications first introduced in the 1950s. After chlorpromazine, known by the commercial name of Thorazine, was approved by the US Food and Drug Administration in 1954, it became an international sensation. This medicine was found effective in treating schizophrenia's devastating symptoms. With ongoing research, antipsychotic drugs have changed and improved in the past three quarters of a century offering those who take them a significantly enhanced quality of life. In addition to tablets, medicines are prepared in liquid form. When staff is concerned that the patient may be storing the pill in his cheek in preparation to spitting it out when no one is looking, antipsychotics can be given as liquid or as a rapidly dissolving oral compound absorbed as soon as it is placed under the tongue. For those who prefer not to have to take daily pills, antipsychotics are available as a long-acting injection that only need to be given every few weeks to every three months depending on the agent. Of course, the caveat is the medicine can only work if the patient takes it!

Another common illness requiring inpatient treatment is bipolar disorder. In this condition patients are manic so thinking, actions and speech are out of control. This disease occurs in cycles with episodes of depression alternating with periods of mania and perhaps with a time of normal mood in between. The mainstay of treatment is a mood stabilizer but medicines like an antipsychotic or antidepressant are added when called for. Manic patients often deny that anything is wrong and proclaim that treatment is unnecessary. Fortunately, some of the newer antipsychotics have the dual effect of treating mania as well as psychosis. The law doesn't allow forced administration of antimanic medicine, but a psychotic state may accompany mania; the law does permit giving an antipsychotic against a person's will so, along with benzodiazepines for their calming effect, the patient can be successfully treated.

Substance use disorders are epidemic. A survey of the demographics of psychiatric inpatients showed that thirty percent met criteria regardless of another primary psychiatric diagnosis such as schizophrenia, bipolar, or depression. Patients use alcohol, opiates, methamphetamine or cocaine; one third tests either positive for or admit to cannabis use. Tetrahydrocannabinol, the chemical in marijuana that makes people feel high, can stay in the body for days to weeks. For people who smoke marijuana once a day or more, urine tests can remain positive for a month or longer.

Medicines to treat chemical dependency are not fully developed. When someone has been addicted to benzodiazepines like Xanax or Ativan, a course of medicine in the same family is given to prevent seizures. If a person has been drinking alcohol to excess, withdrawal is forestalled by monitoring their clinical state and giving benzodiazepines as required for protection against seizures. Inpatients can be prescribed Gabapentin, a medicine already approved for a variety of indications and now used to address the symptoms of alcohol dependence by exerting its effect on brain chemistry. They may also start Naltrexone or Acamprosate to prevent cravings for alcohol or Disulfiram to discourage drinking. Once begun in hospital, these medicines must be continued after discharge for maximum effectiveness.

Opiate withdrawal can last for days to weeks and pose a barrier to patients engaging in treatment if their goal is to leave and use drugs. There are several approaches to treating symptomatic patients while hospitalized. Medications are given that help lessen symptoms of withdrawal such as clonidine, methocarbamol, ibuprofen, and promethazine. Alternatively, patients can start on low-dose methadone, so they experience the benefits of opioids which discourages abandoning the hospital due to withdrawal and forgoing needed medical or psychiatric care. If interested in taking buprenorphine or methadone to help with future cravings, these medicines can be started while the patient is hospitalized with the goal of securing close follow-up after discharge.

The pharmacist's clinical work includes overseeing and advising the pharmacy needs of the sixty-six inpatients. Some are exceptionally difficult to treat; she works with the treatment teams to try to find one effective medicine or a combination of drugs to address the problem. By reviewing all discharge prescriptions and coordinating care with outpatient providers, she helps facilitate a smooth transition when it is time to leave the hospital. This is especially important when medications are prescribed that require close monitoring such as long acting injectables, diabetic treatments, and clozapine, an antipsychotic that requires frequent laboratory tests whose results need be within certain parameters to avoid serious complications.

The pharmacists' work doesn't end with patient care. They lecture at the School of Pharmacy, supervises pharmacy interns and teach medical students and residents the science behind the clinical basics of prescribing medications for the mentally ill. Their immediate work with inpatients is vital, but teaching activities are equally important so that the profession will be enthusiastically carried on by future generations of pharmacists.

(12)

Therapies to Foster Life's Skills

With contributions by Nicole Geise, OTR/L; Kathleen
Kannenberg, ORT; and Lacey Munoz, CTRS

Hospitalized patients have the benefit of occupational, physical, and recreational therapies. Resources are scarce: a small number of providers must serve a large number of patients. Through individual and group treatments, the therapists—whose roles at times overlap—work to improve function and feelings for preparation to face life after discharge.

Other important modalities designed to help individuals cope with emotional difficulties by means of creative expression include art, music, dance and drama therapies. Sadly, because of today's financial limitations, Harborview cannot provide these helpful treatments.

Occupational Therapy (OT) as practiced today is not necessarily to produce the ability to have gainful employment but has the more modest goal of helping a patient succeed at daily activities: attend to personal hygiene, successfully interact with others, and discover "occupations" defined as meaningful activities. Therapists help patients regain the life they want to live before they were ill.

The history of OT dates to the late nineteenth century when physicians identified the need to reform overcrowded psychiatric asylums that offered confinement rather than cure. Physicians found it beneficial to help those in their care find satisfaction in a structured day and benefit from training for a useful occupation. So, in 1917, the National Society for the Promotion of Occupational Therapy was formed. The goals of the organization were advanced by Scottish psychiatrist David Henderson (1884–1965), who noted that mental disorder produced demoralization and hopelessness when someone lost the ability to adapt their activities for successful daily life.

Harborview's two psychiatric occupational therapists provide service on the less-restrictive inpatient units. Here the majority of patients are sufficiently stable so that they can actively engage in treatment. When a person arrives on their unit, the therapist reviews the medical record and assesses whether they are likely to tolerate a brief discussion as to how OT can be helpful. The therapist will want to know what their lives are like: How do they care for themselves, what occupies their time, what activities are meaningful? If they have lost touch with their interests and abilities, the therapist tries to identify the obstacles that have gotten in the way. Are previous resources gone or have cognitive abilities declined? The therapist wants to help the patient find a path back to regain what they've lost or, if that is not possible, to do their best with what they now have.

In addition to meeting with individuals when time allows, the therapist leads groups. These are designed for relaxation as well as for problem-solving. Some struggle with their daily routines at home where they are often isolated from social connections. In OT

groups, patients are advised to recognize the value of having structured activities each day along with identifying the importance of
rest, good sleep habits, self-care, and leisure, a topic shared with
the therapeutic recreation therapist.

In OT groups, patients are encouraged to advocate for
themselves.

*Jimmy is a 35-year-old man who has struggled with his diagnosis of
schizophrenia for the past decade. He's been in and out of hospitals
with distressing frequency. He has often forgotten to take his pills
and he has refused an injection of the long-acting formulation of
his medicine.*

*In group settings, Jimmy was usually reluctant to speak. He'd sit
and quietly listen as others described their troubles and their wishes
to improve their life. After several days, Elliot, another patient about
the same age as Jimmy, described his similar difficulty of staying
on his medicine; this struck a familiar chord.*

*Jimmy spoke. "I don't like the medicine the doctor gives me. It
makes me dizzy and, after taking it, I feel kind of dead. I don't like
shots, so I only want pills...just not the ones I'm supposed to take."*

*Elliot said, "I bet you never told your doctor about this. You
need to tell him so he could give you another medicine that wouldn't
make you feel so bad."*

*It hadn't occurred to Jimmy, usually too shy to speak up for him-
self, that he could ask his doctor for a change. He rehearsed what
he would say and received support and encouragement from Elliot
and the rest of his group. After hearing that others shared the same
experience, Jimmy looked around—and smiled for the first time!*

The therapist provides enjoyable sensory projects such as listening to music, playing bingo, doing trivia puzzles and making

soap. Therapists recognize that people learn better when they are engaged in an activity they enjoy.

Although there are specially trained hand therapists who work with the majority of patients with upper extremity injuries, OT skills are called upon as well.

Lianne, a 21-year-old woman with schizophrenia, heard a voice commanding her to stab her parents. To avoid acting on this terrifying demand, she used the knife to sever her own hand. Lianne's parents, devastated by the horror of what their daughter had done, begged the surgeons to attempt to reattach the hand. Lianne was hospitalized for months, first on the surgical service, then, when stabilized, transferred for continued care on psychiatry.

Lianne's psychosis gradually diminished, and she began to feel hopeful about the future. As a sign of improvement, she was able to comply with the exercises prescribed by OT. Her recovery, not totally complete, took months. Eventually, she returned home to live with her parents who supported her continued psychiatric and medical care. After a year she had regained some movement and she and her parents were pleased with how far she had come. With return of motion, her mood and outlook improved as well.

In preparation for discharge, the therapist assesses each patient's ability to function, looking at how they can care for themselves. Will they need help in managing daily life? Can they find solutions to the problems they will face? Can they cope with taking medicine on their own? If needed, the therapist gives the patient a "Mediset," a plastic pill box divided by the days of the week and times of the day to aid in keeping to a schedule. Therapists administer the Allen Cognitive Level Screen, a test that consists of lacing on a piece of leather according to directions then being able to later replicate the assignment. Although simple in design, this test evaluates the ability to make decisions, function independently, safely perform basic skills, and learn new tasks.

Other tests are used to determine if patients with dementia or depression need extra help after leaving the hospital. One assessment is the Rivermead Behavioral Memory Test, used to gauge ability to remember faces and objects. Can they hear a story then remember the details? Are they able to keep track of appointments by using a calendar? The answers to these questions aid in determining the level at which a patient functions.

The occupational therapist also helps prepare patients for life outside of the hospital. Preparatory tasks include creating a daily routine, considering how to feel productive and thinking about engaging in social interactions. The therapist provides resources to find work or makes a referral to the Division of Vocational Rehabilitation (DVR), a part of the Washington State Department of Social and Health Services. DVR helps prepare a person to get and keep a job by means of counseling, training, and individualized plans.

Physical therapy, the specialty designed to improve physical function, originated in ancient times when physicians recognized the benefits of massage and hydrotherapy. In the modern era, wartime wounds and debilitating illnesses such as polio commanded the attention of physical therapists, who organized into an official organization in the mid-twentieth century so they could respond to the rehabilitation needs of the injured and disabled.

Harborview's physical therapists work with psychiatric patients when they need help to regain use of injured arms or legs. Necessary to success is the willingness to do prescribed exercises so that function improves. Success, though, isn't always possible.

LH is a 41-year-old man with the diagnosis of borderline personality disorder and methamphetamine use. His history includes multiple self-harm behaviors and unprovoked violent actions. His case manager and psychiatrist describe repeated attention-seeking behaviors such as flailing his arms while staggering then collapsing with complaints of having hit his head and demands to be taken to the emergency department "for an x-ray."

LH was hospitalized on the psychiatric intensive care unit after a suicide attempt by running into traffic. His gait was persistently unsteady, and he had repeated falls. Physical therapy was consulted to help him stabilize while walking. The therapist provided LH with an aluminum walker that appeared to be helpful. Unfortunately, this had to be taken from him when he got into an argument with another patient and swung his assistive device at his peer and then at the staff when they attempted to remove it from him. Security officers were immediately on the scene to take away his "weapon" and escort him to his room.

The walker was deemed unsafe, so staff suggested that physical therapy provide a wheelchair. This worked well until LH used the chair in an attempt to knock down a vulnerable elderly man then, as staff tried to secure the chair, he turned it over on himself.

The physical therapist was now at a loss, having exhausted all options for ambulation assist. Conclusion: Not every patient can be helped.

The Department of Psychiatry at Harborview is fortunate to have one recreational therapist. This professional's task is to use activity-based interventions to improve patients' cognitive, social, and emotional function.

The services of recreational and occupational therapy overlap but certain evaluations remain in the realm of one or the other.

Assessing "community integration"—the ability of the patient to function outside of the hospital—is a focus of recreational therapy. The therapist accompanies the person on an outing off hospital grounds and observes the patient's reactions to the stimulus of being outdoors, reactions to strangers, and how activities are negotiated. Can they read a bus schedule and identify a bus stop? Can they safely cross the street?

Arlene, 21 years old and experiencing intermittent periods of depression that are severe enough to require hospitalizations, became partially paralyzed as a result of a car crash when she was 19. She has recently acquired a battery-powered wheelchair so, in addition to helping her with other skills, the recreational therapist takes Arlene into the community for practice. Before each outing, Arlene is asked if she intends to bolt away from her therapist as she has a history of eloping from the hospital and attempting to harm herself when she is away from her normally vigilant care providers. As Arlene's mental state has improved, she can assure her therapist that she will stay close.

Arlene has learned skills from the occupational and physical therapists, but it is the recreational therapist who helps implement these accomplishments. Arlene practices navigating curbs, trying a transportation route where her chair can be accommodated, and practicing other safety measures in the community where the environment is more chaotic than in the hospital. Arlene is a success!

The recreational therapist performs a community safety evaluation with patients who are able to be off their unit. The therapist uses a twelve-block radius to assess how mobile the person will be when out of the hospital and evaluates their ability to read signs, obey traffic lights, and competently cross the street as well as showing willingness and ability to ask for help in case they get lost.

Recreational therapists identify activities that are appropriate for patients with physical limitations as well as for those who have a mental health diagnosis. They rely on services offered by Seattle Parks and Recreation near the patient's home so they can provide a selection fitting to age and ability.

Occupational, physical, and recreational therapists perform important services. They, like social workers, are generally viewed by patients in a positive light. They don't prescribe unwanted medicines like doctors nor are they like nurses who insist on taking them. These therapists are appreciated by those who receive their assistance as making the hospital stay more bearable if not actually pleasant. With the help of the therapists, patients can appreciate knowing that life outside of the hospital will be more manageable and meaningful.

13

The Peer Bridger Program

With a contribution by Nancy Dow

Initiated six years ago, the Peer Bridger program was launched with a two-year grant from King County. This approach has since gained wide recognition for its success at reducing hospital costs and improving the lives of those who use its services.

The Peer Bridger program was created because "business as usual" of discharging patients, often to the streets and without support or resources, was not working—many individuals returned repeatedly to the hospital. An inpatient stay is the most expensive mental health treatment and, when used without absolute indication, it can divert scarce mental health care funds from other, less crisis-focused services.

As a community-based outreach project designed to provide short-term support, Peer Bridgers offer hope, choice, and companionship on the path to recovery. They provides a variety of services as patients transition from hospital care to the community. The program is staffed by "peers"—those who have lived through the experience of mental illness, substance use disorder, or both.

Peer Specialists are fully trained professionals in the Peer Bridger program. This individual self-identifies as someone who has battled with their own illness and has had a successful, if not perfectly smooth, recovery. In the interest of helping the clients with whom they work, they are willing to disclose their course of pain and chaos to their current satisfying and stable life. They are willing to reveal their history because they know that their story will help peers in their own recovery process. To a lesser degree, they may, when appropriate, share their background with staff where the patients with whom they work are hospitalized.

The Peer Bridger program assigns Peer Specialists to each of the three inpatient units to collaborate with medical teams and engage with patients. In visits, they try to smooth patients' angry feelings at being held against their will. They discuss the need to continue taking medicine after leaving and encourage creating a safety plan if things are difficult or go wrong in the community. All they can do is raise the issue of drug use, illegal or otherwise, and remind them of how methamphetamine or too much alcohol gets them into trouble. Still, they are well aware that it takes more than a reminder to inspire someone to change their dangerous ways.

The Peer Specialist helps facilitate discharge and may, if needed, drive or otherwise accompany the person so that they arrive safely at their destination. Usually, the Peer Specialist works with the client for one to two months after discharge but may do so for longer if needed. These professionals assist in locating resources such as food and clothing and, if the patient is determined to remain out-of-doors, the Peer Specialist has been known to go shopping for a tent.

Teddy, a homeless man, had been admitted to the psychiatry ICU six times in three years. His reasons for admission are usually similar: His basic psychotic disorder, normally manageable with his running monologue of delusions, becomes fueled with methamphetamine and causes him to explode. Brought in by police, his violence reaches a sufficiently scary level requiring ICU care for his and everyone else's safety.

Gradually, as the drug clears from his system, Teddy becomes calm and somewhat remorseful. Generally, after a few days' hospital respite, this morose and fairly dignified man is ready to leave and return to living on the street. Social work usually offers a list of shelters which he invariably refuses as "too confining, too dirty, and too many bugs."

Teddy's last hospital stay was in mid-winter when Seattle's days and nights are wet, cold and often verging on snow. This time, Teddy's Peer Specialist came to the rescue. She presented him with a tent and sleeping bag...and Teddy was seen smiling for the first time ever!

Needs are great for a person discharged to the street with no money, means of transportation, food, or items that are usually taken for granted like socks and underwear. Choosing where to start is a daunting task. Peer Specialists have a small budget of funds to buy sleeping bags and waterproof pads for those who are set on living "rough." With permission to shop in retail stores like Goodwill, Peer Specialists buy a stock of items like jackets, ponchos, and gloves. Basic needs are met for a client for about $100.

Lost identification (ID) cards, vital for obtaining basic services, is a perpetual problem for those who live on the street. The peer specialist knows what must be done. To start, the Department of Health and Human Services issues a $5 voucher that the Department of Labor honors to supply a replacement ID. Unfortunately, this process requires the recipient to have a mailing address at which to receive the ID. If homeless, the peer specialist directs the client to Compass Housing Alliance, an organization that provides housing, shelter, and support to people with no place to live. Mail is received and kept for the client with no address.

Clients sometimes lose their Electronic Benefits Transfer (EBT) cards that need replacement, too. Used in all states since 2004 and functioning like a debit card, this electronic system allows the holder to authorize transfer of federal benefits to a retailer to pay for government-approved food items. The program formerly known as "food stamps" has been replaced by the Supplemental Nutrition Assistance Program (SNAP). SNAP benefits are available on the EBT card. Non-food items like cigarettes and alcohol are not available but some fast food chains will honor EBT cards, providing the bearer with the treat of a warm meal.

When Peer Bridgers first started, their motto was "With a bus pass and a cell phone, we can save the world!" Although only a dream, transportation and cell phones are still important supports. Peer Specialists have the use of a car to drive their charges to medical and psychiatric appointments. When ready, clients receive a bus pass so that they can show independence and travel on their own. A Peer Specialist explains:

"I think we've all been in scary situations but that's the exception rather than the rule. We use our own judgment about the level of safety we need to attend to, and we assess how comfortable we feel with each client. We've been trained not to put ourselves in harm's way.

I have clients I will only meet in a public place and won't drive with them in the car under any circumstance. I won't drive with some on a given day if I see that they're agitated, psychotic, or intoxicated. I have started out with a passenger and have had to

*quickly decide that the situation could become dangerous so stopped
and had to ask the client to leave the car. Fortunately, situations
like this are quite unusual."*

What was the most frightening event for this Peer Specialist?
"When a client swallowed a handful of pills while a passenger
in my car."

Peer Specialists stay in contact using pre-paid phones, an especially important resource if the person is homeless. The inexpensive
phone has the peer specialist's number programmed in so the client
can call in an emergency. It would be unsafe to wander through a
homeless encampment looking for the person in need of service,
so the phone is used to arrange for a safe meeting place for the
client to be picked up and driven to their destination.

The Peer Specialist keeps track of when the patient's initial
appointment is set after discharge. Knowing that it is important
to not feel alone as the recovery process begins, they collect the
client from where they are staying, drive them to their meeting
and either stay with them as they are being evaluated or wait until
they are done so that they can be driven back.

The Peer Specialist will do whatever they can to provide support and encouragement. They recognize that it is stressful for
a person just out of the hospital to enroll in an outpatient program and go through the intake process. Sometimes appointments
are scheduled for initial evaluation, but some are on a first come,
first served basis, often necessitating a long wait before their turn
arrives. This is physically and emotionally draining for a person
just a day out of the hospital and now sleeping on the street and
having difficulty in finding food. It would be easy for a patient to
simply leave and totally abandon the idea of outpatient care. The
Peer Bridger program was originally developed to prevent patients

from falling through the cracks. Everything possible is now done to connect clients with ultimately helpful outpatient services.

The Peer Bridger program is designed to provide services that are empowering. For example, in the past the Peer Specialist would drive in a state-supported vehicle to take a person grocery shopping. By doing this, they decided that this activity wasn't geared to foster independence. Now state cars are used for other purposes and the peer specialist accompanies their client on the bus so the person can learn about what route they must use to get back and forth to the grocery and figure out how to buy only what they can manage to carry home. It is hoped that at some future time, the patient can independently tackle and take pride in a successful grocery shopping excursion.

Housing options are a task for members of the Peer Bridger program other than the inpatient Peer Specialist. Although settled in housing and following an outpatient care program, a client may still be in the thoughts of his original Peer Specialist.

The Peer Specialist recalls: "I had a client who was a double amputee and living on the street in a wheelchair. He now is in supported housing and, when I drive past his building and see him outside, I feel that he is one of our outstanding success stories. He knows that he can still reach out to me and call if he ever has the need."

The role of Peer Specialists is shaped by firsthand knowledge that people can recover from the effects of mental illness. Their training and attitude are based on a rehabilitation model that focuses on a person's strengths more so than their deficits. Peer Specialists look for and usually find, small victories for patients in a challenging, often discouraging environment.

14

Consult-Liaison Psychiatry: Care and Support for the Rest of the Hospital

by Taylor M. Black, MD

Since its introduction in 1922, Consult-Liaison Psychiatry, in its early form, was a hospital service designed to assist medical and surgical physicians' care for their patients' emotional and social problems. In 2003, the American Board of Medical Specialties officially recognized "Psychosomatic Medicine" as a sub-specialty of psychiatry. In recognition of the collaborative nature of the work, the name was officially changed to Consult-Liaison (C-L) Psychiatry in 2018. Since then, psychiatrists have bridged the gap between patients needing medical and psychiatric care. "Consulting" psychiatrists aid and advise the physician requesting their service. "Liaison" psychiatrists provide formal and informal education and support to the physicians and nurses of the requesting team. In addition to clinical services, psychiatrists participate in research projects and training of their specialty's future practitioners.

The consulting psychiatrist must understand a variety of medical and surgical disorders and their relationship to abnormal emotions and behaviors. In addition, the consultant needs familiarity with medications and therapies for patients with accompanying complex physical conditions.

Training for consultation psychiatry is intense and long. Physicians obtain a medical degree followed by a four-year psychiatry residency then complete an additional year of fellowship. Some physicians go on to further education in specialized areas like cancer treatment, cardiac conditions, organ transplant, women's mental health, HIV care, and in the interdisciplinary treatment of pain disorders. Maintenance of C-L board certification requires performance reviews, continuing education, and examinations at regular intervals to demonstrate up-to-date knowledge and skills.

Harborview Medical Center, a 413-bed hospital, employs five psychiatrists who either attend full-time or spend a fraction of their work hours on the C-L service. Additionally, trainees from the realms of medical school, psychiatry, psychology, and social work invest weeks to months learning the field. The service also has its designated social worker, clinical nurse specialist, and substance abuse intervention team. Approximately twenty consults per week are requested; the patient in need of consultation is seen by a team member within thirty to ninety minutes of the call for service and is often followed periodically during hospitalization or until the clinical issue has stabilized or resolved.

Physicians rely on the consultant's expertise for a variety of problems. Patients may have a combination of medical and psychiatric illnesses, with each one complicating the treatment of the other. For example, a psychiatric condition can arise because of a medical illness such as a profound depression in the face of a serious or even terminal diagnosis. Patients with pre-existing paranoia or delusions may misinterpret medical care or testing as a threat. An existing cognitive disorder cause by dementia or a traumatic brain injury can disrupt the medical or surgical treatment the primary team deems necessary. In some cases, the team may ask if a patient is malingering or if symptoms are genuinely related to an emotional state.

A member of the patient's primary team calls a C-L psychiatrist, who asks specific questions to determine a need for a consult. Often the reason for the call is related to a vague recognition that there is something wrong, and the consultant must help put this information in context before a clear, actionable question emerges. Sometimes this can be answered on the phone, making a formal consultation unnecessary or the consultant may decide it best to pay a bedside visit to the patient.

> *Ms. L was a 58-year-old woman with a long history of recurrent infections of the skin of her lower legs, related to swelling and poor circulation from heart failure. Because of homelessness, her hygiene and self-care were limited. She denied having the diagnosis of schizophrenia and refused any recommended treatment. Staying in a women's shelter in downtown Seattle for years, she was difficult to engage in social support services due to paranoia. She had occasionally been legally detained from trying to leave the hospital when her infectious symptoms were life-threatening. She refused certain medications on the basis of associations with their names ("'Haldol' is from Hell and I won't take it.") On one visit from her surgical team she removed the dressings on her legs and threw them in the trash.*
>
> *The patient's medical team appropriately identified mental illness as an obstacle to adequate care and called the C-L team to discuss the case. Ms. L was well-known to them from years of hospital*

admissions, and the consultant and primary physician develop a care plan by telephone. Ms. L didn't warrant involuntary psychiatric medication as she was neither sufficiently ill nor a danger to herself or others. The C-L physician recalled that she generally becomes hostile when psychiatrists attempt to speak with her, so an in-person visit was deemed unhelpful. However, she would speak with nurses who could gain enough of her trust to encourage her to accept at least some medical care. Because of nursing support, she agreed to allow the social worker to arrange a post-discharge follow-up visit with a wound-care clinic near her shelter. She left the hospital, promising that she would keep her appointment and the smile she gave as she dressed in a new outfit from the donation closet, gave those who cared for her reassurance that she will really keep her promise.

A consult is rarely called at a patient's request, and often the patient isn't aware that a referral has been made. When the psychiatrist arrives, it is the patient's choice and right to engage in an interview or not. Although privacy is respected, the case must nonetheless be discussed with the requesting team and, if needed, the consultant will contact family and friends familiar with the person prior to hospitalization to gain insight into history and current behaviors and needs.

After the initial visit, patients may be seen on subsequent occasions. If someone is severely injured and spends months recovering on various hospital wards, then a continuous relationship with the behavioral health team is made whether it's with the psychiatrist, psychologist, or social worker. Continuity of care is critical to recovery.

Consult psychiatrists discuss everything with patients from practical decision making to existential dilemmas that may cover how to adapt to grievous injuries and why it is worth going on with life. Meetings are not psychotherapy, which is a long-term process, yet seeing a patient once in the moment of critical need can surely have the same elements of support and exploration.

Some questions asked of the consultation team are more easily answered than others. A common request is for help with managing acutely agitated patients. Such patients can be angry about their medical treatment. They are hostile to care providers and show their rage by yelling and threatening those around them. It's not uncommon for the doctor or nurse to be the target of a physical attack or to be pelted by a thrown object. Patients might pull out their IVs, try to leave the hospital, and generally interrupt medical care in ways that could be dangerous. They are often not making rational decisions about their behavior. For safety, patients may be physically restrained or given sufficient medication to help them calm.

Mr. B is a 34-year-old man with diabetes, and a chronic foot infection. He was hospitalized for a worsening foot ulcer that may need an amputation. He has a long history of distrusting physicians, though he selectively allows some to examine and treat him. He tends to be verbally hostile with nursing staff, makes demands, and will often walk off the hospital ward when upset. Sometimes he returns intoxicated with stimulant drugs that cause even more paranoia and agitation. On one occasion, he accused the nurse changing his dressing of "trying to put something in my wound to hurt me" and kicked his nurse's arm, then tried to roll his wheelchair to the elevator. Security staff and behavioral nursing specialists arrived to restrain Mr. B, and psychiatry consultants recommended medication and started the process for involuntary detainment to keep Mr. B safe.

Another common request is to evaluate a patient who appears unaware of their condition or what is going on around them in the midst of a serious illness. Infection, organ failure, and metabolic derangements can cause our brains, like any other organ, to function abnormally. When delirious, there is an interruption of complex mental operations like reasoning and planning as well as basic ones such as arousal, visual perception, and language. Delirious patients are impulsive and, because they cannot process information, can behave in ways disruptive to their own care as well as being at risk for harming those trying to help them. Delirium also heralds a dangerous state that, if the cause is not found and the condition untreated, could result in death. An important task for the consult psychiatrist is to decide if the patient is truly delirious, a treatable condition, or if the problem is dementia, a chronic and usually progressive impairment of thinking that may be worsened by being in the unfamiliar surroundings of the hospital.

Ms. D is a 76-year-old woman admitted for a hip fracture. She lives in an assisted-living home and her staff describes an increasing frequency of falls. Her family describes memory changes, with difficulty recalling appointments and names, and being confused as to how she should organize her day. They now handle her bills, and she relies on others for meals .

Ms. D had surgery for her fracture and then returned to the ICU. The next afternoon, she asked the nurse, "Where are we going?" and later pulled out her IV before trying to get out of bed unassisted. She told the psychiatrist that "we're all in a tin can ship" and is concerned about the "lizards" she sees on the walls "getting in the controls." The psychiatrist diagnosed delirium in addition to underlying dementia, recommended reassessing her medications, protected sleep time in the ICU, a one-on-one observer for safety, and additional physical therapy and visits with family until she recovered.

Over the next two days, she was increasingly more oriented and alert, and soon proceeded to a rehabilitation facility closer to home, with the suggestion to follow-up evaluation in a dementia clinic once medically stable.

The consult psychiatrist is called upon to evaluate and manage the suicidal patient because they have tried to end their own life and might still want to do so while in the hospital. Suicidal behavior takes many forms, from fantasy to planning to rehearsal to action. Those with self-destructive wishes may practice self-harm or use drugs or alcohol to decrease their inhibitions. Sometimes suicidal behavior is more impulsive, but there is always a story behind the act itself. The most important variable in the outcome of a suicide attempt is method. Ninety percent of medication-overdose and other self-poisoning attempt patients survive, though sometimes this necessitates ICU-level care; using a firearm is the most lethal means of suicide —of self-inflicted gunshot wounds to the head, only 2% survive—while burning, cutting, and stabbing injuries fall in between. Any suicidal act or any person with desire and intent to die warrants a full safety evaluation by a psychiatrist. Thoughts and behavior to end one's life are often symptoms of a mental health disorder or a socioeconomic problem that will respond to support, treatment, and time for recovery.

Mr. A is a 33-year-old man with a history of childhood abuse, chronic anxiety, alcohol use disorder in recovery, and borderline personality disorder. He is the father of a one-year-old daughter who lives with her mother and has recently been involved in a custody dispute. He relapsed to alcohol after a stressful court deposition and used a small-caliber handgun he had obtained in the previous month to shoot himself, directing the bullet under his chin. This caused a fractured jaw and severe injuries to his sinuses and face, requiring an extensive surgical procedure to clean and close his injuries.

The first safety evaluation was in the ICU shortly after surgery where he was still sedated. He couldn't speak clearly due to his tongue injury but expressed relief that he was alive and that he missed his child. He grasped his doctor's hand, opened one eye and was able to whisper, "Thank you."

As he recovered, he began to consider the consequences of his act but still asked to leave the hospital to "sort things out." His willingness to make a safety plan was shaky but, after discussing details with the psychiatrist, he was willing to remain in the hospital and transfer to the psychiatry ward to further explore his experience and to work on a safe and reliable plan for after hospitalization.

Since Harborview serves a high-needs population with scant resources, the primary team may turn to the consultant to help solve complex socioeconomic issues that get in the way of discharge planning. Patients often need considerable coordination both inside and outside of the hospital for management of the psychiatric illness compounding their medical condition.

Ethical questions arise that need clarification and response from the consulting psychiatrist. Can a patient make a decision under the stress of a current medical condition that he would be likely to make if he wasn't so ill? Physicians want to help patients maintain autonomy but, if it seems that decision is made under the influence of clouded and distorted thinking, then it is deemed responsible and ethical to intervene. To help with deciding on a course of care, the medical team, with the aid of the team's social worker, seeks advice from a close relative or, if such a person cannot be found—as is often the case with the homeless—a former care provider or friend is sought to presume what they believe the patient's wishes would be under circumstances of health and clear thinking.

If need for a decision is less urgent, the palliative care service staffed by physicians, nurses, and social workers is called upon to weigh in. Their task is to provide the best quality of existence for a patient at the end of life. Additionally, a decision-making guardian can be sought, and the hospital ethics team can also be asked to help with clarifying the ethical dilemmas and choices. For example, if a patient says that he wants no treatment and just wants to die, is he expressing the wishes he would have made under a less acute situation, or were his wishes made in the moment as he's finding his current level of pain, stress, and fear acutely intolerable? Is an operation or medical treatment advised as a life-saving measure such as the repair of a ruptured aneurism or the beginning of dialysis for kidneys that no longer function? It is the task of the consultation psychiatrist to evaluate the patient's capacity to decide for himself or, if deemed unable to make such a decision, then they offer an opinion as to whether the operation or intervention should go ahead in order to save the patient's life.

A consult psychiatrist described the case of JD, a fifty-four-year-old man who had a progressive neuromuscular disease and was slowly losing the ability to breathe on his own:

'As the consultant, I met JD about a month before he died when he was essentially confined to the hospital. Whenever he'd have a respiratory issue, he would need to go to the intensive care unit. When his situation became dire, his breathing required support by a mechanical ventilator as emergency treatment. He would improve,

and the tube could be removed. This scenario would repeat every few days. We kept asking him, 'Is this truly what you choose? Do you want us to save your life by putting a breathing tube in? Would you want a permanent breathing tube?

Because of this man's neurologic condition, a permanent breathing tube would been a life-sustaining treatment option. Sadly, JD held to his delusion that he could cure himself without this particular medical intervention. He had been coping with this illness for years, and had worked out, for his own mind, a detailed explanation of how he would save himself when the time came. He also let us know that he was okay if he wasn't ultimately rescued by our medical intervention. Nonetheless, throughout his hospital stay, he was unable to engage in a realistic discussion with psychiatrists. And it was obvious that when we tried to clarify his thinking, he would become increasingly distressed. It was clear that our decision-making process was negatively affecting his quality of life.

Eventually, we came to see that what we were doing to prolong his life was only causing this patient more anguish. Psychiatry's intervention was to develop a plan with the intensive care team so that the next time an emergency arose, the patient could exercise his autonomy and decline invasive medical treatment. The discussions we had near the end of his life, acknowledging that his delusion was not an obstacle but an expression of hope and resilience, clearly brought him comfort. It was during one of our talks that I saw him smile for the first and only time. I felt that I'd connected with him. We stopped the fight to insert the breathing tube that he didn't want. We could see that he was comfortable choosing to let his life end, and he died made comfortable by medicines and in peace.'

When patients have attempted suicide but survive, they are hospitalized on a medical or surgical service for care. Suicide attempts take many different forms such as overdose with pills, hanging, self-inflicted gunshot wounds to the head or to another body part or setting themselves on fire. The more violent suicide attempts can occur while the patient is intoxicated, and the most severely injured patients are transported to Harborview as the main trauma center of the region. The few patients that survive their injuries are seen by the psychiatrist as soon as they are able to speak and hopefully benefit from the visit of the consult specialist.

There is an ongoing debate in the psychiatry consultation world about what are appropriate boundaries in discussions with a patient who has had a suicide attempt. This can be a critical moment to talk about essential questions of life and death. The consultant speaks about what could change in their life. The patient is encouraged to develop a safety plan and look forward to a time when they might be less depressed.

Consult psychiatrists try to help the patient understand their underlying motivation for the event and assess immediate safety but the longer-term consequences are often handled by psychologists working with the burn or rehabilitation teams as care progresses.

Another role of a consultation psychiatrist is to help other doctors and nursing personnel understand some of the ways that their own responses to patients can contribute to problems. Everyone is human; everyone has emotions and, for better or worse, everyone reacts to difficult situations. A challenge for staff is to acknowledge that they dislike, are angry at, or even hate a patient. Such thoughts and feelings can cloud judgment. Without meaning to, professionals can inadvertently express powerful emotions in ways that have a negative effect on patients and on themselves. On the other hand, doctors and staff may want to rescue a patient from their behavioral choices that affect illness or reinforce patterns of dependency. This, too, can be bad for both patient and professional.

The C-L psychiatrist helps sort out these feelings to the benefit of all involved.

The psychiatric signs and treatment complications of HIV/AIDS is another area in which consult psychiatrists can be helpful. This illness not the death sentence, but it still remains dangerous and challenging. Adherence to medication can be difficult for anyone but is one of the most critical variables for maintenance of viral suppression. HIV is adept at mutation; any period of time on partial treatment, or off treatment, runs the risk of breeding viral particles that will be resistant to medicine once restarted, making ongoing treatment less effective. This problem makes addressing comorbid mental health conditions critically important as common conditions such as anxiety or depression can affect a person's motivation and compliance necessary to maintain effective treatment. HIV care was one of the first settings in which a consultation psychiatrist was embedded in a medical clinic at Harborview and remains so to this day.

One of the most underserved areas in medicine is that of the classically "psychosomatic" illnesses, formally called "hysteria" and "hypochondriasis." Today, patients are recognized as having "illness anxiety disorder" or "somatic symptom disorder," which are legitimate, generally accepted diagnoses. They have bodily manifestations of emotional troubles with medically unexplained symptoms involving their neurological, cardiovascular, or gastrointestinal function, and often causing pain, low energy, low mood, chronic worry, and insomnia. Having a chronic problem is hard enough; when you hear repeatedly from doctors that there is either no condition at all, or it is "all in your head," and with no specific treatment, this can become a crisis. Unfortunately, patients with ailments for which there is no identified pathology are difficult, if not impossible, to treat. Because of their history of negative experiences with medical care, patients can neither establish rapport with their physician nor can they accept appropriate supportive—and potentially helpful—treatment. C-L psychiatrists can explain these conditions to other physicians and staff, creating a calmer and more accepting atmosphere of care.

Psychiatrists who provide consultation to hospital physicians and staff offer valuable service. They help explain and suggest management for patients with troubled feelings and difficult behaviors. They are ready around-the-clock to aid all who ask for their help and are an important member of the Harborview team.

⑮

Social Work for the Consult Service

With a contribution by Cindy Delamaza, MSW

The role of the solitary assigned social worker for the consult service is about as demanding as any in the psychiatry department. Collaborating with the sizeable team of physicians, nurses, trainees, psychologists, and others involved in patient care, the social worker carries the caseload of the entire service. Between twenty-five and thirty-five patients are in the care of this professional.

As a specialist who works in close proximity to the medical and surgical teams, it is important to be familiar with their language. It makes for better communication to know about diseases, treatments and the shorthand these non-psychiatric providers use with each other. They also need to be aware of the psychiatric manifestations of conditions they treat such as the depression that might accompany cancer or psychosis caused by drugs for Parkinson's disease.

A consult social worker was visiting with a middle-aged man, hospitalized for repair of a fractured leg. His resident physician, in his first year of training, believed that the patient was having panic attacks as manifested by anxiety and difficulty catching his breath. Sufficiently savvy after years of psychiatric work, the social worker, familiar with the diagnosis of panic, could alert the psychiatrist on the team who confirmed that the patient's symptoms didn't correspond to panic but was likely a more serious problem of medical origin. The patient then had the appropriate studies, which led to the diagnosis of pulmonary embolism.

An important activity for the consult social worker is involvement with ethical quandaries. A patient may have cognitive limitations caused by dementia or be delirious and disoriented from a number of causes. When the patient is rejecting what is deemed a necessary treatment such as an amputation for a gangrenous leg or refusing to take in enough food and fluids to sustain life, an ethics consultation is called, frequently inspired by the concerns of social work. The social worker is often the advocate for an ethics committee consultation when they recognize that it would be in the best interest of all concerned to present a dilemma with no obvious good solution to a neutral committee for recommendations.

Although they cannot make a daily visit to every patient, the social worker is aware of each case's needs and directs their efforts accordingly. The entire consult service holds morning and afternoon meetings where coffee and donuts accompany the review of every patient. The social worker is the team member who researches the person's history, keeps track of the dates the patient must appear in mental health court, and contacts family and explores finances. Today's hospital stay can be brief, thereby limiting the time available to make good, solid plans and identify useful resources.

The consult service social worker arranges behavioral health care to follow the medical or surgical hospital stay. The medical social worker is unlikely to be familiar with mental health resources, especially in the more distant parts of the region such as Alaska or Montana. If mental health hospitalization is needed, it is up to the social worker to locate an available bed in the community and to check insurance status, formidable tasks that hold no guarantee of success.

Multiple contacts must be made while the patient is still in care. If permission is granted, family and friends are called to discuss options for living arrangements. Case managers and outpatient providers are asked to help with coordination of care. They are invited to visit to determine if the patient is at a baseline level of functioning so that discharge is a reasonable choice.

With an ongoing bed shortage that never seems to improve, the medical service feels pressure to clear a bed for the next patient who needs one. Some medical providers are inexperienced with patients' mental health needs. Sometimes the medical service chooses to discharge a patient before an experienced psychiatric provider would consider the patient ready. The consult social worker along with the primary team brings to their attention the patient's readiness to return to the community with the lowest possibility of needing repeat hospitalization.

If there is an outstanding legal issue at time of discharge, it's the social worker's task to contact police. According to one social worker:

'We see patients on repeat admissions. DL, a 46-year-old man admitted once again for treating the abscesses he gets from injecting heroin, was ready to be released from the hospital. He frequently has thought of killing his former girlfriend and her two adult sons. DL has never actually harmed this family, but we still have to call police to initiate a 'Duty to Warn,' meaning that the police notify the potential victims that the possible assailant will now be free in the community.

Seattle Police know DL well, having had multiple encounters with him in the past. On one occasion, an officer arrived to speak with him, was assured that he had no immediate intent to kill anyone and spoke with him kindly about how he could deal with his outstanding warrant for arrest for an unrelated crime. She told him, "You're better off taking care of your medical troubles rather than going to jail.'

Arranging for discharge is fraught will all sorts of problems. Social work found this case particularly challenging:

CN is a young woman with borderline personality disorder from Alaska who, in a suicide attempt, burned a large portion of her body with oven cleaner. She spent weeks in the Harborview Burn Unit. Trying to arrange for services for her in Alaska was particularly demanding as she had, so to speak, "burned her bridges" with Alaskan care providers; they were reluctant to resume responsibility for this erratic woman who was so frequently close to killing herself. Even the medical air lift service called to return her home was anxious about carrying this unpredictable and emotionally dysregulated passenger on their helicopter.

The most distressing cases faced by the social worker and the rest of the consult team are the children who try to end their lives.

The social worker relates:

Although infrequent, Harborview's pediatric unit care for children when there is no bed availability in the region's facilities for children with psychiatric needs. We've seen a child of eight who tried to commit suicide and, even more limiting, is that there are only two hospitals, Seattle Children's and Spokane's Sacred Heart who accept children under 13. The patient may have to wait for an available bed for a long time, making it hard on the child, the family, and all involved in their care. Without established pediatric psychiatric care, the child gets the best medical care and emotional support that can be given, but this is far from ideal treatment.

When a patient is ready for discharge, it is up to the social worker to try to cobble together an aftercare plan that might work. Residential options are extremely scarce. When no other possibility exists, the social worker provides options like a list of shelters. No one wants to send a vulnerable person to the street. Working with whatever resources are available, the social worker is committed to finding the best choices for the patient in need.

16

Support from the Medical Consultants

With a contribution by Grant Fletcher, MD, MPH

All sixty-six patients hospitalized in Harborview's three inpatient units have severe psychiatric disorders; often, these are impacted by serious medical conditions. In some cases, illness is immediately evident while in others chronic ailments complicate the picture. Although their conditions might have been previously diagnosed in outpatient clinics, many allow their physical needs to go untreated, ignoring instructions to take medications and follow-up with return visits. Some remain unaware that anything is wrong in spite of distressing physical symptoms.

Because patients may struggle with reality distortions caused by psychosis, intense depression, or disorganization accompanying drug and alcohol use, medical concerns easily become secondary. Abscesses from injuries or injection drugs go unheeded. Blood sugar in diabetics is unchecked until the patient is found unconscious on the street with high enough levels of sugar in their system to make death imminent. Raised blood pressure, chest pains, and abdominal complaints are incidentally discovered in the hospital where patients finally get needed evaluation and treatment.

Hospitalized patients can quickly decompensate with sudden loss of consciousness, difficulty breathing, or chest pain. These are emergencies. A "code blue" is called or the Rapid Response Team arrives on the spot to administer emergency measures and the Medical Consult Service's (MCS) physician soon follows. That physician determines if the patient can remain on Psychiatry for continued care or if immediate transfer to a medical team is warranted.

The MCS is vital for patients hospitalized on Psychiatry. Twenty-five years ago, physicians providing service to patients either in-house or directly concerned with hospital treatment were not as yet an organized group. They have since become recognized as "hospitalists" with their own organization. Fifteen years ago, Rachel Thompson, MD, is credited with creating the MCS as part of the Division of General Internal Medicine. In addition to serving as consultant, the twenty-five full- and part-time hospitalists at Harborview care for in-hospital patients not assigned to a teaching team, evaluate patients before surgery, triage requests for in-patient admission and, as "nocturnists," respond to calls consultation throughout the night.

A single attending physician assisted by a resident and medical student provides daytime staffing for the entire week. Psychiatry interns also participate in order to become familiar with the medical problems their future psychiatric patients might face. Consults to the MCS are mostly requested from inpatient psychiatry and the large trauma, neurosurgical, and general surgical services. Consultants see five to six patients a day including new referrals and visits to those already under care.

MCS is called for concerns about common problems such as untreated wound infections caused by accidents before admission or smoldering urinary tract infections now producing symptoms or hypertension that's getting out of control and requires medication additions or adjustments. Diabetes is a particularly common condition and non-compliant patients will neither check their blood sugar levels nor take prescribed pills or insulin injections. By the time they are ready to leave the hospital, achieving and maintaining tight blood sugar or blood pressure control may not be realistic. Harm reduction rather than perfection is the goal: values acknowledged as "Harborview good," mean the best that can be achieved. To encourage the patient to take medications after hospitalization, physicians prescribe the least complicated regimen.

MCS often sees illnesses that are complex on their own and made more complicated by psychiatric conditions. Heart and respiratory abnormalities abound, creating challenges in treating angina or difficulty breathing from a lifetime of smoking. A catatonic or depressed patient may lie immobilized for days, making them prone to blood clots in their legs that can then travel to the lung. These clots must be treated with blood thinners to avoid death from a pulmonary embolism. And patients will sometimes refuse any medical care which, according to law, can only be forced if refusal endangers the person's life.

Patients over sixty-five are treated on all psychiatric units. They are hospitalized with conditions common to older age such as dementia or they suffer from chronic schizophrenia, bipolar disorder, or excessive substance use. Unfortunately, both the number and intensity of medical conditions increase as people age. The specialized geriatric consultation service is called on for care.

Medical consultant Dr. Grant Fletcher recalls a challenge he'd faced:

I was involved with caring for George, an older man with a history of mania now complicated by dementia. His kidneys failed possibly because of prolonged lithium use and he needed dialysis, which he adamantly refused. We faced an ethical dilemma: Should we force dialysis against this man's will in order to keep him alive or allow him to die which would surely happen if he wasn't treated. The hospital's team of ethicists met with his physicians and his family and, for many reasons, it was decided to proceed. Treating against the patient's will turned out to be unnecessary. At the last minute he changed his mind and agreed to being dialyzed, which was the best outcome possible.

Fletcher also remembers:

Over the years we've attended patients who have had cancers diagnosed while on inpatient psychiatry. There was a woman who'd had an x-ray of her shoulder and the incidental finding of a lung tumor was seen in this film. Another, hospitalized for psychosis, told us that she knew she had breast cancer and wasn't going to let anyone do surgery, radiation or give her chemicals. She believed that the cancer would eventually be cured by the "magical spirit" that protected her.

And we've certainly had some unusual patients in our care. We've been called to see 'swallowers,' personality-disordered men and women who choose to swallow objects like razor blades or pencils. We respond to the psychiatry service's urgent call when this happens. We assess the situation, order x-rays, and call the gastroenterologists to remove the object with their instruments and, if they can't safely accomplish this, then the surgeons are consulted to remove the item in the operating room. Of course, we hope this will never happen again but, inevitably, that's a false hope. Swallowers just keep swallowing.

Whatever problems they face—simple or complex, challenging or routine—the MCS provides an invaluable service to Psychiatry and plays an ongoing role in helping maintain and improve patients' physical and often-delicate mental health.

The Law and Psychiatry

With contributions by Richard Miller, LICSW and Anne Mizuta, JD

It has taken centuries to arrive at today's system of civil commitment for persons with mental illness. Before the creation of asylums, such individuals were considered dangerous and sent to the prison or poor house to be kept hidden from the public and, without treatment, they could be held indefinitely. Even with the establishment of public and private institutions in the nineteenth century, few patients would volunteer for hospitalization. As a result of such a system, a family could put away an unruly relative on a whim.

In the twentieth century, states amended their commitment laws. Individuals now had legal protection to preserve civil rights by being granted a trial with attorney representation before institutionalization against their will. With further changes in the 1950s, the National Institute of Mental Health advocated for streamlining the process to remove unnecessary legal roadblocks.

Two main principles serve as the basis of civil commitment. The first, *Parens patriae*, Latin for "parent of the country," refers to English common law that assigns the government responsibility to intervene on behalf of those judged incapable of acting in their own best interest. The second related principle, "police power," requires the state to consider the welfare of its citizens; this may come at the cost of restricting liberties of those who would otherwise choose to be free. Behind the laws and the physicians charged with following them, are ethical duties to the public and respect for patient autonomy.

Washington, like all other states, has civil commitment laws with strict criteria for when to hospitalize a person against their will. With the total adult population of 5.8 million, there is an estimated 200,000 men and women in Washington with severe mental illness. Many are sufficiently ill, so when hospitalization is advised, they are unable to decide the best course of treatment for themselves. In these cases, the state steps in to protect the patient and to consider the welfare of the community.

Involuntary hospitalization is based on at least one of three criteria: (1) a person may be deemed a danger to themselves by actively attempting to end their own life or by put it at risk by a dangerous act; (2) a person may be considered unsafe if they attempt or threaten to harm property or other individual; (3) a person is considered "gravely disabled" if they cannot provide for their own needs of basic safety and health. One cause could be that a someone's cognition might have sufficiently deteriorated, thereby preventing them from receiving essential care or being able to care for themselves. In order for an individual to be hospitalized, the relevant criterion must meet the condition of "imminence," implying that calamity is likely to occur in the near future.

A person in need of evaluation is referred to a Washington state-employed designated crisis responder (DCR). This trained professional meets with the individual and gathers collateral information from police, care providers, and/or friends or family who have witnessed distressing behaviors. Interviews help determine if involuntary hospitalization is indicated. Anyone can become an affiant and call the DCRs whether they are a medical or mental health provider located in the emergency department, in another hospital or in a clinic. Any citizen can call the DCRs if they believe that the person is at risk of harming themselves or another or they noted bizarre, disorganized, or dangerous behaviors.

The Involuntary Treatment Act focuses on people with mental illness, but as of April 1, 2018, Ricky's Law addressing substance use disorders went into effect. Now, community members who are a danger to property or themselves or others or are gravely disabled due to a drug or alcohol problem may be involuntary detained to a secure withdrawal management and stabilization facility.

Ricky's Law is generally not invoked at Harborview. Most patients considered for detainment suffer from mental illness alone or, if they struggle with substance abuse, it is usually combined with a mental disorder and not an isolated diagnosis. In any event, there are only a limited number of available beds designated for chemical dependency treatment; about forty are located in eastern and central Washington and none are in Seattle.

If detained by the DCR, the initial hold lasts for seventy-two business hours and, to the consternation of the detainee, holidays and weekends do not count. Not all patients can be assigned hospital placement. Unfortunately, beds are at a premium everywhere. In the event the patient must remain in the emergency area, they are placed on a "single bed certification" meaning that some degree of basic mental health treatment is provided during the waiting period. Technically, this qualifies as "boarding," an undesirable situation defined as when emergency department evaluation is complete and the decision has been made to either admit or transfer the patient, but there is no available bed. Unfortunately, this plight can go on for hours to days.

If the patient isn't ready for a safe discharge as the seventy-two hours draws to a close, physicians and the court evaluator, under the direction of an Involuntary Treatment Act program manager, are sent to assess the patient's condition. If the court evaluator agrees that hospitalization should continue, they submit a request for a hearing in front of a Superior Court judicial officer asking to extend the stay to fourteen days. The patient can agree to remain on their involuntary hold to continue treatment or they can request release by asking for a hearing at King County Superior Court. A public defender is assigned, although, on rare occasions, an individual will choose to represent themselves. The first hearing is after the seventy-two-hour hold is about to expire, wherein the institution requests that the patient be held for an additional fourteen days. As that time reaches the tenth day and continued hospitalization is indicated, then the hospital files for a hearing for a ninety-day commitment.

At Harborview, in-person hearings are rare. Video court, established as a system that is more humane than in-person court appearance, has become routine. Patients from other hospitals in King County who used to be transported to Harborview for their hearing no longer have to undergo the stress of travel by ambulance or van. They once had to wait, possibly in restraints, for their case to be heard in front of the judge. It's kinder for patients to be able to remain in their own therapeutic environment and those at Harborview follow the same procedure, being removed from their treatment setting for only the duration of the trial.

Video court is a formal, legal proceeding. The patient, his or her attorney, and the prosecuting attorney are in one room while the judge is located elsewhere; all see each other on television screens.

The court evaluator argues for the hospital and call witnesses to bolster the case. The patient, too, has the opportunity to request witnesses on their behalf to demonstrate why further hospitalization is unnecessary. The court relies heavily on substantive, first-hand evidence; therefore, the court evaluator supports their case by offering the medical record written by physicians and staff who observe daily behaviors. If the patient was brought to the hospital after being seen acting in a dangerous manner such as running into traffic or assaulting someone in the community, it would be insufficient to merely read a police report; actual witnesses must come to court to testify. If the judge decides to prolong the hospital stay, the decision is based on "a preponderance of evidence," a standard of proof used in civil trials meaning there is a greater likelihood than not that the case brought by the prosecution proves their version. It is then up to the defense attorney to attempt to discredit the evidence and show that the prosecution's argument does not support their allegations.

Court can be tense for all concerned. Families, friends, and even case managers are stressed as they suffer through the patient's crisis. They may be ambivalent about having to testify about events prior to involuntary hospitalization, knowing that they are doing so as a caring person but against the patient's wishes. Likewise, hearings can be extremely stressful for patients. It is disconcerting for a patient to have to listen to family or case managers publicly describe them at their worst moments. They have often been without medications for the twenty-four hours prior to the hearing, as they have the right to refuse being medicated so that they can be free of side effects and alert enough to participate in their own defense, which can lead to being unpredictable in court. Patients can be distressed enough to lash out, so security is available to keep everyone safe.

To help ease the tension, Harborview has Murphy, the placid chocolate Labrador, as the official court comfort dog. Murphy is teamed with Senior Deputy Prosecutor Anne Mizuta. After completing training, they now work as a therapy team in which Murphy is licensed to share his calming presence with witnesses. When not working, Murphy, wearing the green vest to which his Harborview picture ID card is attached, spends his days napping on his bed under Ms. Mizuta's desk. Welcoming pats and occasional snacks, he brightens the days of staff, physicians, and visitors who stop by to greet him.

Not every case is guaranteed to be decided in the hospital's favor. After hearing the prosecutor's information, the judge can choose to dismiss the case, believing the evidence insufficient. Or, even prior to a hearing, the prosecutor may feel that the case for commitment is too weak and couldn't withstand the evidence offered by the defense. So, a hospitalized patient can go free. This may happen even though everyone may believe it is in the best interest of the person to remain in hospital, but these are legal proceedings and clinical opinion is trumped by the requirement to follow the law.

In spite of several weeks of treatment, the patient may still be in need of continued inpatient care, so the court is petitioned to extend the stay for to up to ninety days. At the hearing, evidence must be even greater than that offered for a 14-day hearing and be substantial enough to convince the judge with a level of certainty that the patient should remain hospitalized. Of course, if the patient is held for ninety days but improvement is seen, discharge can occur within that time.

When a ninety-day hearing is proposed, the patient has the right to request that their case be heard in front of a jury rather than as a bench trial with the judge alone deciding the case. This event would take place in the King County Courthouse in front of a jury selected by the same system for all courtroom trials: A pool of potential jurors is called from the community and, with the patient present, the prosecutor and public defender make selections based on who they think will be most advantageous to their side of the case.

A jury trial is a complicated process that can require the services of many and take days to complete. The patient is transported to and from the courtroom by ambulance and is accompanied by staff at all times. As in any jury trial, proceedings begin by the lawyers and judge determining what is to be allowed in the hearing. Physicians, staff, police, community members, and family may be called as witnesses for both sides. As in all trials, the patient as defendant is offered the chance to speak on their own behalf, an opportunity usually declined.

For a patient to request a jury trial is unusual; perhaps only a half dozen have been carried out over the last decade. When it happens, though, this is a major event with an often-unpredictable outcome. As in any trial, the jurors make the call. Rather than a determination of guilt, the call is to continue hospitalization or to discharge the person from care.

LK, originally from Russia, had been in the US for the last ten of his 45 years. His English was adequate, his beard and hair were long and unwashed and how he managed his life when not in hospital was unclear. Because police would find him sleeping under a bridge or in an abandoned house, they would bring him to Harborview because they observed him talking loudly with invisible demons and he look like he hadn't eaten in a long time. After several previous psychiatric commitments, he seemed to disappear when released, never keeping follow-up appointments made on his behalf.

During the current hospital stay, L continued to speak to unseen demons, reluctantly ate his meals and even more reluctantly took medications. By the time of his 90-day hearing, he wanted to leave the hospital with no particular plan other than returning to the bridge under which he was often found.

L told his lawyer that he wanted the jury trial to which he was entitled. Nurses trimmed his hair and beard, encouraged him to bathe and shampoo, and dressed him in the brown tweed suit supplied by his lawyer. For four days L rode an ambulance to court, accompanied by his nurse. In front of the jury, his lawyer made the case that he had the right to live as he chose and that he harmed no one by doing so. The prosecutor argued that he was brought into the hospital as thin as a skeleton, floridly psychotic and had no capacity to provide for his own basic needs. The jury, siding with the patient, felt otherwise and the judge set him free to return to his chosen lifestyle.

Risking a decision made by a jury is every patient's right.

JB, a retired professor of accounting, was 78 years old and suffering from rapidly advancing dementia. His wife could no longer care for him at home because of his aggressive outbursts and neglect of his person and surroundings. She brought him to Harborview as a place where he could be safe.

JB repeatedly asked to go home. He didn't want to be anyplace else and certainly not in the care facility found for him by his social worker. When his lawyer asked if he wanted a jury trial for the hearing that could potentially commit him for an additional ninety days, he said that this was his best chance at leaving the hospital and agreed.

And so, Mr. B had his days in court. The trial, including jury selection, lasted three days. Witnesses were called for both sides.

The public defender, Ms. D, found a distant relative who said that he could stay at her house. Witnesses for the prosecution spent much time in explaining dementia to the jury. Mr. B's wife appeared as one of these witnesses and, in tears, told the jury how painful this experience was for her as she had to argue against her husband's wishes to return to their home where she felt unsafe in his presence.

After both sides completed presenting their case, the jury deliberated for several hours and, not having come to a conclusion, their deliberations resumed for several more on the following day. In the end, the jury decided to recommend continued care for Mr. B. Since a ninety-day commitment means a transfer to the state hospital, he would go there when a bed was available on the Older Adults' unit. Mrs. B cried as did his public defender who told her and the physician who cared for Mr. B that she was doing the best job she could as a lawyer carrying out her client's wishes.

All lawyers in ITA court are licensed by Washington state. They have been trained in both criminal and civil law and have had considerable experience in these areas before assuming their current roles. Harborview has eight full-time ITA prosecutors who carry a large and sometimes overwhelming roster of cases, all of which need absolute attention as well as several dozen public defenders who work for four separate offices in King County.

A public defense attorney is assigned to provide representation at no cost. Rarely, the patient will decline this attorney's services and has the right to represent themselves. Even more rarely, the patient is successful at convincing the judge to decide on release. There are also times when the patient is unable to communicate their wishes to their attorney, so a professional *guardian ad litem* is appointed to represent the person's best interests. The public defender's task is to support and defend the rights of the patient and represent their client's wishes in court, even if that may not be in the patient's or the community's best interest.

Prosecutors and public defenders are mindful that protection of civil liberty is at stake; for example, if there is a case involving threats of using a firearm, the prosecutor will consider the consequences of civil commitment in that the person will lose the right to possess a firearm indefinitely unless a court restores that prerogative in the future.

The ITA process and its court have a special place in the legal system. Lawyers need to be familiar with mental health diagnoses and treatments in order to have the best understanding of the clients with whom they work. The goal of all involved is to see the patient become healthy and make sure that they are given the best opportunities in life while civil rights are preserved.

18

Chemical Dependency:
Inpatient Assessment and Treatment

With contributions by Matthew D. Iles-Shih, MD, MPH;
Jared Klein, MD, MPH; and Jessica Warmbo, MHP

The general impression today of many healthcare professionals is that they see mind-altering substances used with increased frequency and taken in greater quantity. In the past, patients would seek care under the influence of marijuana obtained by illegal means or with a card "certifying" medical need. Now, with the advent of marijuana's legal status in Washington state, as many—if not more—patients present as intoxicated from recent use. In addition, alcohol and stimulants continue undiminished as popular substances of choice.

Harborview cannot offer inpatient treatment for those who are addicted to substances, as this requires a specialized facility and staff. The hospital and clinics do provide assessment and outpatient treatment for those who want to try to be free of dependency. Hospitalized patients are guided to the path of recovery as they are encouraged to connect with groups where they can find help after discharge.

In recent years, Harborview has developed several services dedicated to addressing chemical dependency. The inpatient consult team for Addiction Services is staffed by a psychiatrist, two internists trained in addiction, a peer specialist, a nurse, a pharmacist and members of a separate group of clinicians, the Screening, Brief Intervention and Referral to Treatment (SBIRT) providers. When called for a consultation by the primary team, this group provides care for a patient ill with a medical or surgical condition who is also struggling with the complications of addiction. The consultants perform a full psychiatric assessment with a particular emphasis on the patient's substance use history.

Ronald, a 35-year-old man who lived on the street, had fallen on hard times when he couldn't find work as a laborer in Seattle. He had initially begun using opioids for a painful back injury that prevented him from even the lightest work. When physicians advised pain management without using narcotics, he obtained the pills he craved by purchase on the street. After finding this source prohibitively expensive, he switched to heroin, an option he could manage to afford.

Since Ronald occasionally re-used unclean needles, he paid the price by developing an abscess that caused a high fever. Frightened and believing that he could now die, Ronald was admitted to the surgical service where his abscess was drained, and his infection treated with intravenous antibiotics. The surgeons saw that he was in the early stages of opioid withdrawal and paged the on-call addiction medicine attending.

Several treatment options were offered to Ronald, who was willing to consider becoming free from his addiction after his recent medical scare. He and the physician agreed on starting Suboxone, a prescription medication used in treating those addicted to opioids that can help patients lead a much-improved life without illegal opioids.

Addiction Services can present a reasonable and acceptable plan to help the patient get through the current crisis and provide a referral for longer-term treatment to be followed after discharge.

Physicians on the team have general certification in the specialties of psychiatry or medicine. After training, they complete a fellowship in addiction medicine then pass an examination to receive subspecialty board certification. Physicians must demonstrate ability to provide screening, intervention, and treatment as well as competence to address the psychiatric and physical complications of addiction.

Three physicians whose time is limited by their obligation to serve in other parts of the hospital, provide part-time service to the Addiction Medicine team. As a result of minimal staffing, they are unable to see all patients in need. One physician on the team estimates that approximately 10% of the total hospital census of 413 beds has an opioid use disorder at any given time and the prevalence of alcohol use disorder is estimated to be about twenty times greater.

After visiting with the patient, physicians make recommendations to the primary team. They may suggest starting or adjusting a currently prescribed medication such as methadone, a replacement therapy for illegal or prescribed opioid addiction, or Suboxone, which contains buprenorphine (a partial opioid agonist, which blocks the opiate receptors and reduces a person's urges) and naloxone (which helps reverse the effects of opioids). Suboxone must be initiated when the patient is already in withdrawal. If started too early, it can trigger symptoms such as muscle aches, nausea, and chills. Suboxone replaces opiates such as heroin, morphine, and oxycodone in the brain, and thereby blunts intoxication and prevents cravings. When used outside of the hospital under appropriate supervision, it has been shown that Suboxone, as a medication-assisted therapy for opiate addiction, lowers the risk of fatal overdoses by half.

A frequent challenge physicians face is to recommend treatment for a patient addicted to opioids and hospitalized after trauma, surgery, or childbirth whose condition is complicated by acute pain. Treatment strategies are complex with the need to find a balance between addressing ongoing addiction and pain relief.

Since patients cared for at Harborview come from a variety of countries and cultures, the drugs they use for altering their mood and consciousness can be quite different from substances taken by those born and raised in the United States.

LO, a 45-year-old non-English-speaking man recently arrived from Somalia, was admitted to the orthopedic service for repair of a complicated arm fracture. His primary team noticed that he had signs of psychosis and his blood pressure remained high, as did his temperature, pulse, and rate of breathing. As with other patients admitted to the hospital, his urine was screened for alcohol and other drugs, but this test returned negative. In hopes of sorting out then treating this man's condition, his doctor requested an opinion from the Psychiatric Consult Service.

The consulting physician was somewhat puzzled. He wondered if there might be some substance used by the patient that wasn't detected by the standard screening test. He asked the physician on the Addiction Medicine service and learned that these symptoms could possibly be caused by "khat," an amphetamine-like stimulant derived from the leaves of the khat tree that grows in East Africa. LO was one of many patients from this region who regularly chewed khat for increased energy, confidence, and a general sense of well-being.

Physicians working on Addiction Services are familiar with a number of drugs used in other countries and carried to the United States. They've seen the effects of *kratom,* a traditional medicinal herb derived from the leaves of a tropical tree native to Southeast Asia that produces euphoria at low doses and sedation and decreased pain when taken in larger amounts. These effects are similar to commonly used opioids. Addiction physicians have seen the distressing effects of *krokodil* from the Ukraine and Russia and they are frequently confronted by other new and unregulated psychoactive substances obtained on the internet.

Funded by special grants, Harborview is fortunate to be able to offer a unique service: the SBIRT team. The history of SBIRT dates to the 1980s when the World Health Organization recognized the need for efficient methods to provide early intervention among alcohol users. Accurate screening tests for alcohol in primary care settings, emergency departments, and trauma centers allowed doctors to help patients recognize and manage their substance abuse problem before it became too late. By 1990, the Institute of Medicine—an independent, non-government group now called the Health and Medicine Division of the National Academy of Sciences—designed the intervention available today to fill the gap between primary prevention and more intensive treatment for those with substance use disorders. Created with the goal of improving community health, this course of treatment was designed to reduce the prevalence of adverse effects among substance abusers. Originally developed for applying to alcohol use disorders, the scope of SBIRT has expanded to include addressing prescription and illegal drug use.

SBIRT consists of three major components. The first element, screening, happens when the team member meets the patient and inquires about their substance use history. The answers to standardized questions determine if there has been accompanying risky substance-related behaviors. Finally, the provider asks if the patient is thinking about change.

The next phase is a brief ten-minute intervention where the provider "requests permission" to "raise the subject" and offers education about risky behavior as it applies to the patient's substance of choice and to increase their motivation to reduce risky behavior. If interested, the provider gives the patient written educational materials they can read at leisure.

Finally, if the patient agrees, they receive a referral to brief therapy or an additional treatment in which the patient could realistically participate.

Alicia, a 70-year-old widowed woman, was a typical patient for whom an SBIRT consult was requested. She was currently being cared for on the orthopedic service where she had had an operation to set her fractured leg. She had been falling at home, sometimes in the living room and, on this occasion, had fallen down the flight of stairs that led to the basement. When she was first admitted to hospital, her blood showed a high level of alcohol.

G, the SBIRT team member, was asked by Alicia's nurse to talk to her about her alcohol use. Before starting a conversation, G asked Alicia if it was all right to raise the question of alcohol. When Alicia agreed that they could go ahead and speak, she told G that she didn't think that alcohol was a problem. "I just have a couple of glasses of wine with dinner. It's not a big deal."

G administered the Alcohol Use Disorders Identification Test, a screening tool used to determine if the amount of alcohol drunk is a problem. As their conversation progressed, Alicia did admit that she also drank during the afternoon when she was feeling especially lonely. At times she thought about drinking less but never seemed able to do so. In fact, she was beginning to drink more, and lately she had begun to start her day with a glass of wine instead of a cup of coffee. She did admit to feeling guilty at needing to drink so much but believed that there was no one with whom she could discuss her feelings even though her niece asked her more than once if she was intoxicated while they spoke on the telephone.

As the conversation progressed, G asked Alicia if it was all right to speak about her possible problem as a result of drinking too much. Reluctantly, Alicia agreed, and G admitted that alcohol had contributed to her troubles, including the broken leg caused by her fall while drinking. Alicia was interested in reading the pamphlets G left for her and said that she'd like to speak further about meeting with the individual therapist for the twelve free sessions available with Harborview's SBIRT team since she wasn't ready to meet others in a group setting such as Alcoholics Anonymous.

The SBIRT team often sees patients who have been heavy users of alcohol, marijuana, or illegal substances like methamphetamine and opioids but don't want to cut down or stop. Rather than trying to encourage a patient to be substance-free, the SBIRT representative introduces harm-reduction strategies. As an example, a patient addicted to heroin is told about getting and using clean needles and educated about having access to Narcan, a substance self-injected or administered by another person, to reverse the effects of having taken more heroin than their system can safely handle.

SBIRT's task is also to offer referral options if a person wants to start or to continue on their path to recovery. Alcoholics Anonymous (AA) and Narcotics Anonymous (NA) may not be to everyone's taste. Groups such as Buddhist Recovery is an organization with meetings that focus on the benefits of meditation and SMART (Self-Management and Recovery Training), a secular and science-based group that offers an alternative to AA, NA and other twelve-step programs. Specialized services such as Seattle Counseling Services exist for those who identify as LGBTQ.

In keeping with SBIRT's attitude of acceptance, they frequently refer patients to Seattle's Recovery Café. This free-standing red-brick building serves as a safe setting for individuals who have been traumatized by addiction and other mental health challenges. Here they can explore housing options, education, and employment as the ultimate goals of maintaining freedom from drugs and alcohol. Chemical dependency is a major issue for many patients at Harborview; it is through these avenues of help that Harborview staff hopes to reduce abuse and reliance on substances.

19

Clinicians Share their Skills

Psychiatrists provide assistance to various Harborview clinics and even to patients outside of the hospital. They offer consultation to other providers and advise on their patients' psychiatric needs. Consultants address complex medical problems and mental health issues that can complicate compliance and response to treatment. A number of Harborview clinicians willingly share their specialized expertise with those who call on their services.

THE PERINATAL CONSULTATION SERVICE

With a contribution by Carmen Croicu, MD

The *Partnership Access Line (PAL) for Moms* is a telephone consultation line for providers. This free service is sponsored by Washington state's King County, which recognized the importance of increased awareness for the mental health problems that arise in the weeks and months surrounding the birth of a child. Any provider can receive consultation, recommendations, and referrals to available resources in their community. Psychiatrists who staff *PAL for Moms* announce their availability by giving talks, sending written material to clinicians, and calling on a "health navigator" who makes the service known in Washington and in other states.

Harborview-based Carmen Croicu, MD, is one of a half dozen perinatal experts in the UW system who offer consultation to a widespread group of providers both local and distant. Croicu and others take turns answering calls received on the perinatal consultation line staffed five days a week during business hours. Calls come from primary care physicians, obstetricians, psychiatrists in private practice, and nurse practitioners in the university system, around Washington, and from other states in the Pacific Northwest. When a complex patient is referred by the Harborview Obstetrics and Gynecology Service, the individual can be seen in person in keeping with the hospital's collaborative care model.

On the telephone, consultants are asked to consider mental health issues for women who are pregnant, are having difficulties in the first year after birth, or are experiencing infertility or loss of a pregnancy. They discuss topics that include psychiatric disorders, complications, or medication treatment. Callers have numerous questions regarding psychiatric medicines for pregnant women or for those considering becoming pregnant and about women struggling with postpartum mental health concerns. For questions too complex for a phone discussion, patients are referred for in-person psychiatric consultation to a University of Washington clinic where they will see a psychiatrist with expertise in maternal health.

Croicu recalls a memorable case:

A provider was treating a pregnant patient with significant bipolar disorder. Without consultation, he decided to stop one of her medicines on his own. As a result, the patient needed emergency hospitalization for becoming suicidal as a result of severe depression. The provider wasn't aware of the consultation line but called after the fact. He was grateful that he need not feel so alone, and he would now have support for when his patient was released from the hospital.

CARING FOR THE INCARCERATED AT KING COUNTY JAIL

With a contribution by Martin Buccieri, PA-C

Videoconferencing in psychiatry is far from a recent innovation. In 1959 the Nebraska Psychiatric Institute introduced long-distance treatment and training. Ten years later, Massachusetts General Hospital provided psychiatric consultations via video at a Logan International Airport health clinic. In the decades that followed, this method of management, now referred to as "telepsychiatry," came to be recognized as valid as in-person care. Telepsychiatry is accurate in diagnosis, effective in treatment, and efficient, as it saves time, money, and resources.

Inmates, just like anyone else, may experience mental health issues while incarcerated. Yet bringing the inmate to a clinic for an in-person interview is costly as well as it creates risk each time the detainee leaves their secure setting, requiring special transportation accompanied by guards. Similarly, psychiatrists and other mental health providers willing to work in jail are few, as an evaluation at the facility carries its own hazards. Telemedicine eliminates the risks and conserves limited resources associated with on-site psychiatric care, yet inmates still have access to mental health treatment.

The first telepsychiatry for the incarcerated was introduced by the California Department of Corrections and Rehabilitation in 1997 and is now an indispensable part of their mental health system and of many others, including that of Washington state.

In a secure and private setting, inmates tell their stories and discuss their symptoms and concerns with the provider on the video screen. Interview times vary from forty-five minutes to an hour according to patient need. Problems are no different from those of patients cared for at Harborview: chemical dependency, psychosis, depression, and mania to name a few. Medications, if indicated, are advised but, unlike inpatients at Harborview, must be taken by the individual's willingness to do so, as they cannot be compelled.

Treatments for inmates differ somewhat from those available to patients at Harborview. If an incarcerated resident is experiencing symptoms of withdrawal from illegal drugs or alcohol, they are referred to medical rather than psychiatric providers. Although some popular street medications may be requested such as benzodiazepines and Seroquel, these are not prescribed except for special indications. If an inmate becomes dysregulated and acts out with violence, they're placed in solitary confinement, a procedure implemented for safety.

Between the downtown facility and the Maleng Regional Justice Center in Kent, the King County jail system incarcerates close to three thousand people at any time. Many inmates have both substance abuse and mental health issues that need medication and therapy. To respond to this significant need, King County Jail contracted with Harborview to offer psychiatric services via telemedicine. Although the Harborview providers can see only a tiny fraction of those in need, they still make their impact in addressing the overwhelming shortage in the correctional system. Two providers, Kelly Panaanen, ARNP, and Martin Buccieri, PA-C, see patients for a total of eight hours each week, doing what they can to take a bite out of this huge problem.

CARE IN ADULT MEDICINE CLINIC: PSYCHIATRY

With a contribution by Taylor M. Black, MD

The Harborview Adult Medicine Clinic (AMC) is a busy primary care clinic staffed by physicians, nurses, pharmacists, medical assistants, and social workers. In addition, it serves as a training site for internal medicine residents, supervised by attending physicians who also carry a caseload of their own patients.

The psychiatrist in AMC attends the clinic part-time, acting as consultant to the Behavioral Health Integration Program of social work therapists who offer patients support, behavioral activation and assistance with solving problems. The psychiatrist is available for case review requested by the clinic's primary care physicians regarding medication and treatment plans. When the problems are excessively complex, the psychiatrist assumes management.

In a typical afternoon, the psychiatrist will see one to two new consultations and about five patients in follow-up. The range of problems varies: schizophrenia, bipolar disorder, traumatic brain injury, personality disorders, substance abuse, PTSD, adjustment to medical illness, somatization disorders, complex anxiety symptoms, and disabling depression. All are complicated by occurring at the same time as medical illnesses. Many patients would otherwise be best served in a community mental health clinic setting with a team including a case manager and access to groups and recovery activities, yet lack insurance funding through Medicaid to access such services.

A psychiatrist recalls a particularly concerning patient where no one medication or combination has been helpful but being invited for a return clinic visit is an important aspect of her care:

CM is a woman in her 60s with substantial early-life adversity including witnessing and directly suffering abuse from caregivers who had mental illness and substance use problems. She has been able to function, work for periods of months, and has raised one child to adulthood, but suffers with lifelong mood and anxiety symptoms. Drinking alcohol runs in the family and is an intermittent a problem for her, leading to personal and occupational difficulties. She has also been in abusive relationships and still has flashbacks to them, affecting sleep and creating ongoing avoidance of public places. She has developed moderate heart failure and diabetes and is now less resilient to the emotional and physical stresses she must face.

When CM does not follow care guidelines, she is prone to ankle swelling and injuries from falls and has been hospitalized twice with complications including signs of cognitive impairment and delirium and a toe that is showing signs of chronic infection and may need amputation.

She has been seeing mental health providers periodically over many years and expects that this will remain part of her treatment plan. However, due to lifelong difficulties trusting others, she tends to cancel appointments when struggling more. Yet, when she does come to clinic, she accepts her prescriptions which she will probably fill and appears pleased with the attention paid to her by the staff and always reminds them that she needs to make an appointment for "next time.".

The patient still firmly believes that her appointment every three months with her psychiatrist is very important and not to be missed and her psychiatrist agrees.

Because a considerable number of patients visiting the clinic have a high rate of behavioral health comorbidity, assistance with mental health concerns are a necessary addition to the medical services offered. These are the invaluable services provided by AMC staff.

CARE IN ADULT MEDICINE CLINIC: THE BEHAVIORAL HEALTH INTEGRATION PROJECT

With a contribution by Michael Wenger, MSW

The Behavioral Health Integration Program (BHIP) started at Harborview in 2007, a time during which the government offered medical but not behavioral health benefits; therefore, a new program was tried: A clinic care manager would work with the primary care physician (PCP) to arrange for the patient to receive evidence-based behavioral health services. The patient now had a team that also included a psychiatrist and therapist, taking the burden of frequent visits focusing on mental health issues from the PCP, who was freed to focus on medical concerns.

Social workers, under the auspices of the psychiatry department, screen patients for conditions such as depression and anxiety then meet with them for supportive or other forms of psychotherapy every two weeks while the PCP or psychiatrist visits with the patient at intervals of months for medication adjustments. The psychiatrist might not actually see the patient in person but offer advice to the prescribing PCP. One of the roles of the social worker is to coordinate this process. The arrangement is supposed to last for six months, but it is acknowledged that not all Harborview patients will fit this mold and care can continue for a much longer period of time until targeted symptoms have abated.

There are two BHIP social workers in AMC—one each in Family Medicine and the Women's Clinic—while others are assigned to clinics off-site. These clinicians carry a caseload of fifty to seventy-five patients. Patients occasionally present with emotional dysregulation and thoughts of harming themselves or ending their lives and clinicians are familiar with how to address these issues. While much work can be considered routine, tense times can occur.

One clinician, Michael Wenger, MSW, recalls:

I've worked with a man in his 50s for several years. Among other serious medical issues, he has end-stage renal disease and needs dialysis three times a week. He's terribly racially biased and it's been hard to sit with him and have to listen to his angry outbursts. I referred him to our special cognitive behavioral therapist who was helpful in examining his prejudices and, as a result, he became far less enraged and listening to him is much easier.

Wenger describes a patient he has worked with for years and will likely continue to do so.

WL, almost 70, has a lot of orthopedic problems and is excessively overweight, a condition complicating just about every aspect of her life. Her complains of unremitting isolation manifested by her inability to leave his apartment except for rare occasions, a problem that hasn't improved even after years of medications and psychotherapy. Our therapy in BHIP should be helping her to develop support and activities but, this treatment, like all others, hasn't worked.

My patient never misses an appointment and always expresses gratitude for the time we spend together. I accept that we're not going to see much change, but I recognize that I'm performing a much-appreciated service by being a reliable part of her medical support network.

MADISON CLINIC

With a contribution by Roger Michael Huijon, MD

For thirty-five years, Harborview's Madison Clinic has been caring for patients with HIV and AIDS. The clinic's internists, infectious disease specialists, nutritionists, pharmacists, researchers, and social workers provide highly specialized attention to all who seek it. Mental healthcare professionals furnish psychiatric consultation that includes recommendations for medications and continued psychological treatment.

The clinic's consulting psychiatrist receives requests to evaluate patients with a wide variety of conditions. In addition to mood disorders, there are many contending with substance use disorders, some of which are accompanied by symptoms of psychosis. Patients can be quite ill, needing to be seen as frequently as every week until stabilized or referred to more intensive care. Many individuals are pleased that they have the Madison Clinic to rely on and, as HIV has become more of a chronic disease rather than a death sentence, patients are seen for years of care. When they need more than intermittent visits with the clinic psychiatrist, they are referred for support in the community.

A psychiatrist recalls:

I treated a man in his 30s diagnosed with HIV about ten years before he started coming to Madison. A transplant to the Seattle area, he had lived with his family in another state before moving here. He also used a fair amount of methamphetamine and his psychosis was probably secondary to taking drugs. He wasn't ready to stop using so it was difficult to control his symptoms.

We had a family meeting with the patient and his partner, and we were joined by his mother in her home state on the telephone.

Our goal was to come up with a plan that would keep this patient safe, sober, and still taking his antiretroviral and psychiatric medications, as he had real problems with adherence. With our plan in place and after making some medication changes, he seemed to be doing better. It's hard to say how durable his improvement will be but, for now, everyone, including the patient, is pleased with his accomplishments.

INTERNATIONAL CLINIC

With a contribution by Zahra Shirazy, MD

International Medicine is a small clinic providing medical care to Seattle's poor and indigent refugee and immigrant populations. Most patients come from East Africa, southeast Asia, and Mexico needing attention to their chronic medical conditions. While trying to cope with the struggles of being transplanted to in an unfamiliar country, having been displaced from their homes, and having lost family and finances, they are burdened with anxiety, depression, and post-traumatic stress disorder as a result of their traumas.

Psychiatrists make an important contribution. Dr. Lorin Boynton established a presence in the clinic twenty years ago and the service she started has grown with a purpose to identify and treat mental illness of patients of different cultures and attitudes. It is important to build trust in people whose lives may have been missing a reliable system of care. With the help of interpreters, the psychiatrist aims to connect with the patient in a compassionate and culturally appropriate manner.

Because of time constraints with the psychiatrist assigned to work one day per week, seeing up to a dozen patients on that day, treatment is limited to medication management. There used to be a clinic psychotherapist but funding no longer permits this service. A specialist in treating victims of torture use to work in the clinic in past years; a lack of funds has also eliminated this important service.

The current psychiatrist, Dr. Zahra Shirazy, says:

Some cases make me feel hopeless. All odds are against them. They escape from the traumas of their country trying to save their own lives then they come here with multiple psychosocial stressors: homelessness, limited resources because of their status. We wonder how they survive.

She goes on to describe a patient she found touching and memorable:

Luz is an undocumented immigrant from Mexico. She has genetic abnormalities that show in her appearance and influence the way she views the world. She went through devastating experiences in her home country, and how she survived them is impressive. Her vulnerability is increased by her multiple medical conditions and her limited treatment options. But she always comes to her appointment with a smile on her face no matter how distressing her situation. At this time, her housing will have to change, and she must move far away from Harborview, the place she considers her second home. The anxiety evoked by this situation is heart-wrenching for me as her provider.

Dr. Shirazy also adds:

My patients are so gracious and demand nothing. They are completely appreciative of their care.

International Medicine Clinic psychiatrists may ask for the services of Community House Calls, initiated twenty-five years ago, which provides home visits to help with issues such as a family member having trouble, difficulty keeping appointments, and other non-psychiatric medical problems that may arise.

The mission of Community House Calls is "to contribute to the well-being of refugee and immigrant patients, families, and communities through a partnership that promotes culturally sensitive care." This is the mission of all who work in International Medicine Clinic. Although resources are at times limited, this is a valuable service to the underserved indigent refugee and immigrant communities, one that will continue to aid these at-risk people.

(20)

Electroconvulsive Therapy: A Last-Resort for Help

With a contribution by Amelia Dubovsky, MD

Harborview psychiatrists offer the option of electroconvulsive therapy (ECT) to patients whose illnesses have not responded to other treatments. ECT involves a brief, controlled electrical stimulation of the brain through electrodes placed on the scalp producing a transient seizure while the patient is under anesthesia. The procedure lasts only minutes. Research supports proven effectiveness, so the popular stigma associated with ECT has been gradually disappearing and its use is now recognized by respected professional organizations such as the American Medical Association and the American Psychiatric Association.

ECT is called upon to address a variety of serious conditions. After failed trials of medications and therapy, severe, unremitting depression has been shown to lift in about three quarters of the patients treated. Additional conditions responsive to ECT include the psychosis of schizophrenia, the mania of bipolar disorder and catatonia, which, if left untreated, can be fatal when the affected patient refuses to eat or respond. This procedure is effective and relatively safe: Even pregnant women suffering from depression can receive ECT rather than using medications whose effects and side effects can put mother and fetus at risk. Patients with compromise hearts can get through their ECT session without problem and enjoy its benefits.

Even though side effects and complications of ECT are few and ECT sessions are usually straightforward, this treatment is not a permanent solution. After the 8–12 sessions generally needed to achieve remission, medications and therapy as well as additional ECT administration may be required to maintain relief.

Administering ECT requires receiving specialized instruction from senior physicians. The supervising physician who oversees the training then attests that the trainee can now work independently. At Harborview, three psychiatrists are certified to administer ECT. The treatment is used for ill inpatients on the psychiatric service and, on occasion, for patients on a medical service too mentally compromised to participate in their own care. Amelia Dubovsky, MD, one of the psychiatrists, attests:

> I think it's the most effective treatment in psychiatry, perhaps besides good psychotherapy. I see results in a week or two compared to weeks to months with medications. I say this because I've seen it: This is the closest thing we have to a miracle treatment, as it works when everything else has failed.

Dubovsky recalls a man whose result was a resounding success:

> TL was in his 70s with the history of a good life with a loving and supportive family, many interests, and a career in engineering which

had always been a source of pride. The problem arose when he retired from his job of forty years and, feeling the loss of identity and foreseeing a dismal future, a profound depression set in. He received trials of multiple medications and had three inpatient hospitalizations, but nothing worked. At home he would remain in bed for days at a time; when eventually rising, he would pace around the house, wringing his hands and refusing to speak to those around him.

Before his most recent stay at Harborview, TL tried to end his life by repeatedly stabbing himself. While recovering from his wounds in the ICU, he attempted to strangle himself with a cord attached to his bed. I have never seen a patient as hopeless as TL.

With symptoms of psychosis compounding his depression, TL's doctors and family were eventually able to convince him to give ECT a try. And he did! After the first week of three treatments, his wife described him as "amazingly improved." After another two weeks of treatments, his family said that he had just about completely returned to his normal self. Even the patient reluctantly acknowledged that he was feeling much better and surprised everyone by saying that he would now consider going fishing with his grandson.

This was an unprecedented response for someone who surely would have died without ECT. Appreciative of his result, TL could honestly admit that he felt like he had been rescued from the depths of Hell.

Not all patients respond to ECT, as they may have an underlying diagnosis that leans more to a dysfunctional personality rather than a mood or psychotic disorder. Dubovsky recalls:

Tamara, a pleasant 20-year-old woman with hair cropped close to her scalp and an array of stuffed animals surrounding her in bed, *had spent most of the previous ten years in institutions. Since early childhood, her life's goal was to end her life. She'd made numerous suicide attempts by overdose, strangling and refusing all food and drink for weeks at a time. At Harborview, she would repeatedly try to harm herself no matter how closely she was watched. She'd made a sharp weapon from a plastic spoon and ripped her pajama top to fashion a noose.*

Tamara had had many courses of psychotherapy and medicines for what was taken to be an underlying depression with psychosis. Nothing worked. As a last resort, she agreed to try ECT. And that didn't work either.

ECT is truly an effective and life-saving procedure for many. There's no guarantee of the results for either the short or long-term, but watching the recovery of patients from depression, mania, catatonia, and psychosis has been undeniably impressive.

(21)

Geriatric Psychiatry

With a contribution by Shaune Demers, MD

Of the 32 million people living in the United States in 2019, approximately 5.8 million suffer from dementia. As the proportion of the population age 65 and older continues to grow, the number of Americans with Alzheimer's or other dementias will also increase. This figure is predicted to more than double in the next thirty years. Unfortunately, there are only about 2,000 specialists in geriatric psychiatry at this time, a number far from sufficient to attend to the needs of this impaired population.

A geriatric psychiatrist trains in general psychiatry in addition to a taking a fellowship in caring for an elderly population. Geriatric psychiatry emphasizes the biological and psychological aspects of normal aging, the psychiatric effect of acute and chronic physical illness, and the medical and emotional aspects of psychiatric disturbances of older age. These specialists work to prevent, evaluate, and treat mental disorders in the elderly as well as to provide psychiatric care for healthy, older patients.

Several Harborview psychiatrists have expertise in working with the elderly. They serve in different areas: in the outpatient Memory and Wellness Center, as consultant to nursing homes and in the main hospital where they see patients staying for brief or longer-term care.

For example, the geriatric psychiatrist in Harborview's outpatient memory clinic meets with patients from the entire northwest region. Referrals arrive from as far away as Alaska and Hawaii when they pose a difficulty in diagnosis or a puzzle in treatment for their local provider since Harborview serves as the region's only tertiary care facility for memory loss. This clinic offers a comprehensive program: In addition to the geriatric psychiatrist, it is staffed by neurologists and internists who focus on the unique problems of the elderly. The senior psychiatrist will, at times, supervise residents and students who are learning about memory care. A geriatric fellow, a psychiatrist who has decided to specialize, may also be a part of the clinic's medical team.

Evaluation is exhaustive. Cognitive complaints, either as identified by the patient themselves or, more frequently, by family or a referring physician, are thoroughly assessed. Complete physical and neurologic exams are carried out and patients may be sent for neuroimaging consisting of a CT or MRI scan to look for brain abnormalities that can contributing to memory loss. Neuropsychological testing, an extensive set of tests done with pencil and paper and performed by a specially trained neuropsychologist, is another means of trying to specifically identify how brain health affects memory, planning, abstract thinking, problem solving and behavior.

Memory loss can occur as a result of various conditions. Many patients seen at Harborview have Alzheimer's or a less common vascular dementia caused by the blockage of small blood vessels in the brain. Patients are usually over seventy years old, but dementia can present in middle-age as well. Some are sent by the neurologist or internist because they are having psychiatric complications of a degenerative nerve disorder such as Parkinson's or Huntington's disease, multiple sclerosis, or amyotrophic lateral sclerosis named after the twentieth-century baseball player and known as Lou Gehrig's disease.

Although uncommon, persons concerned that they are beginning to lose their memory will request an evaluation on their own initiative.

TK is a 57-year-old cardiologist who comes to clinic because he's concerned that he is becoming increasingly forgetful. At times, he is unable to recall his patients' names or conditions. He describes difficulty remembering to pay his bills and is concerned that his office practice is declining. Dr. K's wife noticed that he appears depressed. Without telling his wife or colleagues, he decided to seek consultation.

Dr. K participated in extensive psychiatric, medical, and neuropsychologic testing. He received the conclusions of the testing— early-onset dementia—with sadness but with equanimity. The psychiatrist offered an anti-depressant and Donepezil, a medication that's prescribed in the hopes of improving memory, awareness, and the ability to function. Knowing that his impairment will likely worsen gave him the opportunity to prepare for his future.

Family members may recognize their relative's decline and initiate the request for an appointment. Many patients, though, will keep the appointment only with great reluctance. Once in clinic, the person's story can be much different from the family's description of events leading to the consultation. Individuals may deny having any memory problems at all in spite of others noticing that they misplace objects, leave the stove burning, or repeat what they say without recognizing that they're doing this. They may neglect self-care, have difficulty identifying the right word to express their thoughts and, when out of the house, have trouble finding their way home. It is their choice whether or not to cooperate with an evaluation. If an individual refuses to participate in a cognitive exam, the psychiatrist tends to believe that they wouldn't do very well if they did take the test.

> *Mrs. D, a 74-year-old woman, was brought to clinic accompanied by her sister who described her as having memory lapses and keeping herself and her home clean. Mrs. D lived in the house she'd shared with her husband and wanted to remain there after his death although she admitted that she felt quite lonely without his companionship. Mrs. D was angry at the suggestion that she might be impaired, saying that she didn't know why her sister brought her to clinic as she was sure that she had no problems that needed attention.*
>
> *Reluctantly, Mrs. D agreed to participate in examinations, believing that if she did so she'd be able to prove her sister wrong. Unfortunately, Mrs. D's testing revealed considerable impairment. She repeatedly used words like "thing" and "stuff" when asked to name objects. She scored well below average in all areas of memory and reasoning. At completion of testing, she was found to have met the criteria for Alzheimer's disease. She was told that it would be both safer and more pleasant for her to change her living situation and move to a home where she could be supervised as well as have the company of others.*
>
> *Mrs. D's sister understood the seriousness of the situation and assured the psychiatrist that she would advocate for Mrs. D to return to speak with the social worker, and that she would ask Mrs. D's internist to encourage her as well.*

The psychiatrist watches the interaction between patient and family. There may be a sense of tension, anger, and fear pervading the meeting. The person may be reluctant to reveal information with others present and the family may be unwilling to provide descriptions of events that would be difficult for the patient to hear.

Today's treatment of dementia is still evolving. Medications give variable results so other modalities are recommended. Those affected are encouraged to live and enjoy their lives as much as possible. They're told, "You're not a different person because you have this diagnosis." They're advised to be socially active and, equally as important, to exercise as evidence has shown that activity can benefit the person's ability to attend to their activities of daily living although it won't slow dementia's inevitable progression.

The psychiatrist particularly seeks to treating accompanying mental health issues such as depression and anxiety. Patients are encouraged to address excessive alcohol or illegal drug use as these will only complicate and worsen already-impaired cognition.

The geriatric psychiatrist, with the assistance of the clinic's dedicated social worker, discuss how the patient will best receive care. This might mean remaining in their own home with the aid of caregivers. The recommendation may be to take advantage of one of the many available day programs or, if more support is required, the individual may be offered full-time care in an adult family home or in a more formal memory care facility. Any of these options can be declined unless there is a legal guardian designated to make the decision in their best interest.

A 64-year-old man was referred to clinic by his primary physician at the request of his sons. They could only describe his problem as "acting strangely." This retired engineer had been active in his church and had begun to make unwanted sexual advances toward women who were either strangers or neighbors he already knew.

On examination he had no memory deficits but substituted words, such as when he was asked to identify a "book" he called it "paper." Other neuropsychologic tests were abnormal as was his MRI scan that showed shrinkage of the temporal and frontal lobes of his brain. After consideration, this man was diagnosed with fronto-temporal dementia, a progressive, untreatable, and extremely debilitating condition. With this knowledge, the patient and sons could consult with the clinic's social worker to help make future plans.

Care providers have recognized needs, too. The clinic provides community resources, referrals to caretaker support groups, and identifies family dementia-friendly activities readily found in Seattle.

Harborview is recognized as having a strong geriatric psychiatry presence, with busy providers on teams working hard to fulfill the growing need.

(22)

Psychiatry Residency Continuity Clinic: Psychotherapists-in-Training

With a contribution by Matthew D. Iles-Shih, MD, MPH

To become a fully trained psychiatrist, residents are introduced to the various techniques of psychotherapy. Starting with seminars and readings, they prepare to work with their first patients. Instruction continues throughout the four-year course. Education never ends but, after passing exams, they qualify to independently treat their own patients if wanting a future practice that includes psychotherapy.

Patients, also called "clients"—a term used to signify de-medicalizing the therapy experience—are referred by other hospital practitioners or request an appointment after hearing about the clinic through outside sources. Those who seek treatment are screened by a senior resident for clinic suitability and by staff for financial concerns. Clinic does not offer auxiliary services such as case management or advice from social work, so patients must have a certain amount of stability and their own access to external support. Acutely suicidal or otherwise self-harming individuals or those significantly impacted by active substance use are referred elsewhere for more comprehensive care.

Therapies are matched to patients' clinical and residents' educational need. Supportive treatment helps clients cope with current concerns; psychodynamic therapy, whether brief or long-term, explores the past to help understand the present; and Cognitive Behavioral Therapy helps patients modify negative reactions by changing how they think about themselves and those around them. Dialectical Behavioral Therapy, taught in an elective seminar, is another form of highly specialized therapy. This treatment, originally developed at the University of Washington and now widely practiced, is designed specifically for those who struggle with regulating emotions that cause destructive and life-threatening behaviors. Residents can modify any technique as appropriate for each individual case. Additionally, trainees may also prescribe medications. And, from the beginning, patients are told that treatment lasts only as long as residency lasts, although there are rare exceptions when the resident-patient relationship continues.

> Dr V, resident in her third year of training, met with HJ, a 25-year-old woman referred to clinic after psychiatric hospitalization at Harborview. This formerly optimistic and productive schoolteacher's life had been disrupted by a manic episode causing her to lose her job, her boyfriend, and her sense of self. Although now stabilized on medicine, she was demoralized as she feared that she couldn't regain what she had lost and that her future would be destroyed by bouts of illness.
>
> Dr V met weekly with her depressed and anxious patient as HJ tried to make sense out of her diagnosis and the fallout that follows from episodes of illness. In the beginning, Dr V used the technique

of supportive psychotherapy, assisting HJ to come to terms with her diagnosis and what it might mean to her future life.

As time passed and HJ calmed, Dr V transitioned to Cognitive Behavioral Therapy, where she was able to engage in a manualized treatment that helped with symptoms of depression and anxiety. Considered successful after twelve weeks, Dr V resumed supportive and somewhat exploratory modes of therapy, which led to HJ returning to both full-time employment and a satisfactory social life.

Five years later, Dr V, now an attending psychiatrist, still meets with her patient every few months for brief supportive "brush-ups" in a unique and helpful connection that has endured for years.

Two further relationships stand out as meaningful to patient and physician alike.

Dr R, a resident-in-training, was assigned to treat LB, a 65-year-old woman with depression. LB was compromised by multiple medical illnesses including a cancer that was rapidly taking her life. Dr R asked his supervisor for advice and received approval and encouragement for his idea of visiting his patient in hospital. Over the following weeks, LB became increasingly ill and passed away. Dr R was tearful in his supervision hour as he reported that his patient's family asked for him to be present at the funeral as his care and support for LB had been extremely important in her last weeks of life.

Dr A, completing her final year of training, began to see GS, a 93-year old woman who managed, with difficulty, to attend clinic from her nearby retirement home. She'd had an active life as a public relations specialist, writer, and politician before age prevented her from engaging in the activities she loved. Dr A's goal was to help her patient accept limitations imposed by age and explore what could provide satisfaction now. Dr A graduated and wanted to transition GS to another therapist, but she became too infirm to attend any further appointments. After discussion with a supervisor, Dr A continued to visit the patient in her care facility. To show how meaningful this outreach was, GS dedicated her final book of essays to the therapist who had become a beloved constant in her life.

Patients are given to understand that their therapist is a psychiatrist-in-training who will be carefully supervised by senior practitioners. Supervision is by individuals and also in peer groups led by an experienced clinician. To monitor progress in both settings, residents present cases for discussion. With permission, therapy sessions might be videotaped, and recordings reviewed with the supervisor in order to assess the subtleties of patient-therapist interaction. Supervisors and residents who find that they work well together occasionally continue their educational connection after the trainee's graduation.

It is indisputable that psychologically well-adjusted clinicians provide the best psychotherapy. In addition to struggles facing trainees in their own lives, therapists react to the emotional upheavals of their patients. To provide support and to help residents gain control and understanding of their own emotions, the training program provides the opportunity to engage in psychotherapy at no cost for six months. Many find this experience sufficiently valuable and continue in therapy after the half-year is over.

Both patients and residents profit from participating in the Psychiatry Residency Continuity Clinic. Patients are able to engage in therapy in spite of having limited financial means. They accept that their therapist is in training but still appreciate the care and concern offered by a professional helping them achieve the most out of their lives. Residents benefit from experiencing their first close relationships with patients and know that they can rely on the support of qualified supervisors. It's everyone's gain.

㉓

Suicide Prevention and Recovery

With a contribution by Kate Comtois, PhD, MPH

Deadlier than traffic accidents and homicide, suicide is the tenth-largest cause of death in the United States. An average of 130 Americans died by their own intention each day in 2018 and numbers rise each year. Since 1999, the suicide rate has climbed 35 percent, although statistics may not accurately reflect the extent of the problem as the stigma surrounding intentional self-destruction leads to underreporting. The estimate of people of all ages who have had suicide attempts and suicidal thoughts are likely to be many times the total of those who have actually taken their own lives.

The problem of suicide strikes close to home. In 2019, 18 deaths per 100,000 people in Washington state were due to intentional self-harm. Seattle/Tacoma has the second highest suicide attempt rate out of the thirty-three largest metropolitan areas in the United States. For decades, Harborview clinicians and researchers have been focusing efforts through education, support and access to care with the goal of preventing loss of life by suicide.

For two decades, nationally recognized psychologist and researcher Katherine Comtois, PhD, has made her goal to give the best chance of success to suicidal patients and to the clinicians who treat them. With the aid of her team, she has developed treatments, interventions, and conducted clinical trials to prevent suicide in populations of diverse ages, cultures, and backgrounds. Her accomplishments not only have saved lives but have improved care and encouraged clinicians to become more comfortable and willing to work with this challenging and demanding patient population.

When Comtois began her work as a post-doctoral candidate in 1992 at the Harborview Mental Health Center, she joined the dialectical behavioral therapy (DBT) program which had its origins in the pioneering work of the University of Washington's Marsha Linehan, PhD. Comtois explored the idea of suicide prevention, vital for patients with borderline personality disorder. She engaged those prone to self-harm in DBT.

In 2005 Comtois was introduced to the Collaborative Assessment and Management of Suicidality (CAMS), a clinical approach used to identify, assess, and manage suicidal outpatients that has shown evidence of effectiveness in resolving suicidality. She believed that this intervention might be a good potential solution for patients who were acutely at risk for killing themselves but who had neither the luxury of time nor the need for a full DBT program.

Comtois describes CAMS as a therapeutic framework rather than a specific kind of psychotherapy, and, in fact, it is a collaborative endeavor between patient and clinician. The therapist sits next to the patient as the assessment form is completed and the treatment plan is arranged with input from both. CAMS is framed so that the patient must keep their focus on their suicidality and explore its underpinnings. The paperwork gives the therapist a working structure as well as strong documentation that they've done everything that there is to do.

The CAMS initial assessment lasts from fifty to eighty minutes. Treatment can begin then, as the course progresses, success is measured by having three consecutive weeks where suicidality is low, and any residual thoughts or feelings can be managed independently. A referral may then be made to another therapist to work with the patient on their underlying mental health issues: depression, PTSD, substance abuse, bipolar or personality disorders. The CAMS therapist might also choose to switch therapeutic modalities and keep the patient under their own care.

Comtois believes that suicide prevention should extend to the locations where it's needed. She and her team bring their efforts to the US military where suicide is a significant concern. Her research and clinical skills are also applied to Preventing Addiction-Related Suicide, a program designed to forestall a person from taking their own life. She's expanded the concept of the "Caring Contact." Patients coping with suicidality are known to be most vulnerable following discharge from the emergency department or from an inpatient stay. It has been shown that repeated follow-up contacts by phone, text, email, postcard, or in-person reduce suicidal behaviors.

Working with suicidal patients stresses providers. It takes a professional comfortable with their own emotions and willing to accept and manage the risk of losing their patient. It can be easy to feel as helpless and hopeless as their client. To address anxiety, it's important to talk with a peer or be supported by a clinical team. The team shares the burden of responsibility with the primary clinician, making it more sustainable to continue caring for those who want to end their lives. It's acknowledged: This work is certainly not for everyone.

Not every patient treated is successful. Comtois describes her case:

CAMS doesn't engage everyone. My patient was a former govern-ment security employee who wanted a career where he would also be able to keep a firearm. He had several suicide attempts, each followed by hospitalization. He hated psychiatry and he hated the hospital. There was no point to try to keep committing him since he got nothing out of his stays. He saw me only because it was a condi-tion of a court order. And nothing worked. He was angry at every-thing and especially at his former wife who wouldn't resume their relationship. His worldview was rigid and inflexible. Eventually, another attempt at taking his own life succeeded. We did every-thing we could, but our efforts failed. We might have had a better chance at keeping him alive if we'd gotten to him before he became so hardened against the mental health system and everything asso-ciated with it.

Comtois gives an example of success:

A thirty-year old man suddenly suffered a painful and irreparable breakup with his partner of five years. He was completely undone by this unexpected rejection. In his CAMS assessment, we were able to identify the key drivers of his goal of suicide. He needed his identity and his life back. In the nine weeks of treatment, we targeted his hopelessness, the feeling most tied to his suicidality. I focused on the idea that one can survive a breakup. I encouraged him to reconnect with work and begin dating. Once he could see his life going forward, his suicidality resolved. Victory!

Although at this time, Comtois prepares to leave Harborview as her base and transfer her clinic to elsewhere in the university, she continues to participate in the Center for Suicide Prevention and Recovery. At Harborview, those she has trained will continue what she has begun in treating this patient population in desperate need of care so that they can live.

(24)

Outpatient Services

With contributions by Sunny Lovin, LICSW;
John T. Blatchford, LICSW, LMHC; and Carolyn J. Brenner, MD

Harborview's Mental Health and Addiction Services (HMHAS), the facility's outpatient clinic located at the Patricia Steel Building, provides for the care of approximately 2,000 patients, the majority of which are insured by Medicaid. An average day sees about 300 patients on the schedule. Although there is no provision for formal walk-in services, clients nonetheless arrive without an appointment to present their concerns and ask for help. Clinicians share triage responsibility so, if people do appear unannounced, they get attention for their urgent needs and have a more formal appointment set for the future.

HMHAS offers crisis intervention, medication management, and various psychotherapies as well as treatment for patients with mental health issues that are complicated by chemical dependency. Supportive employment and housing teams aid in providing comprehensive care.. In addition to therapeutic meetings, clients participate in cooking, nutrition, and art activities, and even an evidence-based mindfulness class. By offering groups, the clinic takes into account the need to address multiple elements that make for a healthy life.

Approximately two dozen mental health practitioners (MHPs) serve the many patients who rely on the outpatient clinics. MHPs are trained in social work and have received their master's degree or are licensed mental health counselors (LMHCs). LMHCs also have a master's or doctoral degree in mental health counseling or in another field relating to issues of the mind. They have completed a period of supervised clinical work and passed a qualifying examination. These clinicians provide brief therapy and case management alone or in combination.

Case managers are their clients' safety net, but this option is available only to patients with Medicaid, the sole payer supporting case management. Case managers assess current needs and assist with identifying housing, food sources, vocational opportunities, accessing community resources, and applying for financial or health benefits. They help plan for crises as they encourage the development of coping mechanisms and setting support systems in place while boosting their clients' strengths.

The role of the outpatient social worker who focuses on community mental health is different from their inpatient counterpart. As care coordinators and point-of-contact for their caseload of fifty to seventy-five patients, outpatient social workers function as part of an interdisciplinary team that consists of mental health practitioners, nurses, prescribers who are either medical doctors or nurse practitioners, peer supporters, and employment and housing specialists.

Serving as the front door to the clinic is the Intake & Brief Intervention Service, known as "IBIS." They provide time-limited assistance to clients referred from within and outside of the hospital. Their task is to make an initial assessment and then extend brief services to people who can then be referred elsewhere if in need of long-term treatment.

To provide care for their large clinic roster, outpatient services are divided into teams with each unit staffed by a case manager, nurse, physician, and nurse practitioner. The three Mental Health Recovery Service teams serve clients whose needs range from the minimal to the most intensive involvement. Teams meet each morning to talk about the day's schedule and try to predict if any safety concerns will arise. Patients are seen with the frequency their individual cases require.

Patients who depend on the outpatient clinic may not be in a stable condition. If their care providers haven't heard from them in a reasonable period of time, an outreach team, another of HMHAS' services, goes to where the patient lives to check to see if they are safe.

In addition, HMHAS also has specialized clinics that operate within the general outpatient setting. Dialectical behavioral therapy (DBT) clinic provides DBT and some cognitive behavioral-based therapies. For patients who struggle with impulses to end their life, the Collaborative Assessment and Management of Suicidality is a therapeutic framework offered by providers specially trained in this life-saving treatment. Geriatric clinic serves patients with dementia or with some special needs not necessarily associated with chronological age.

Clients with severe mental illness often have accompanying medical issues. Unfortunately, their psychiatric state can prevent them from seeking needed care. To address this problem, a primary care nurse practitioner has been integrated into the structure of the clinic so patients will now be shepherded through laboratory tests and given help with making and attending medical appointments.

An important element of HMHAS is the Addiction Service. In the past, this service encouraged a very traditional model of abstinence but now has modernized its treatment approach. Providers are certified by Washington state to work with individuals experiencing problems with substance use, abuse, and addiction. The Addiction Service offers a full spectrum of care options including harm-reduction advice and intensive outpatient programs. Staff aims to meet patients at their current state of wanting help. If they're willing to reduce their use of substances but are not ready to abstain, that's fine. If they're amenable to joining a 12-step program, that too is appreciated, as is the willingness to try Suboxone or other medical treatment to eliminate cravings. This flexible approach has proved more successful than the rigid attitudes of former times.

The clinic offers a setting of stability for clients. It serves as a place to go where they feel accepted. The drop-in center provides a comfortable atmosphere where coffee and breakfast are always available, and bingo and movies help pass time. This is a welcome opportunity for people who may not have stable housing or ready access to food. The center offers a sense of community to all who seek it.

Clinic Director Carolyn Brenner, MD, has been associated with HMHAS for a decade. She finds it rewarding to work with people with severe mental illness and appreciates the ongoing connection she maintains with her clients. Here she can develop a relationship where they come to trust their physician. "Since I've gotten to know a patient over years," she explains, "I can tell when something isn't right. I can see that they're struggling, and we try to intervene early before things get too bad." She appreciates watching her patients progress from their psychotic state in the hospital to returning, after discharge, to independent living, taking their medications, working at a part-time job, and generally feeling better.

Dr. Brenner recalls a patient she'd worked with over the years who was an outstanding example of success.

I started seeing Anna when she was in her mid-twenties. She wasn't taking any medicine, was staying in shelters, and hadn't spoken with her family for years. She would be kicked out of places like grocery stores because she would talk to herself and, at times, would yell and make a disturbance.

Underneath it all, I knew that Anna was a sweet person. She scared people but she was just as scared herself. Over time she came to trust us. Eventually, she was willing to accept medicine and keep her appointments. She worked on social skills: not yelling and making eye contact. Progress was slow. Things really turned around when we were able to get housing for her. As she gained insight, she could tell me how scared she was when she heard frightening voices. Eventually, she told me how lonely she felt.

Anna and I spoke about how much she wanted to make friends and she did what she could to accomplish this. Eventually, she confessed that she would like to have a romantic relationship. She met a man with whom she formed a connection and she contacted the family whom she hadn't seen for years. They now got together for holidays and, when Anna finally married, the family hosted her wedding party. It was so nice to see Anna reach her goals.

With melancholy, Dr. Brenner remembers other patients whose stories had a sadder ending.

Once a year we have a memorial service for patients who have died in the previous year. The case managers and the Department of

Spiritual Care organize a memorial service. We invite clients, staff, and faculty who might want to attend. We hold this in our drop-in center as we come together to remember anyone who was lost in the last year but focus on the clients we've lost in our mental health center, our community. Death often comes more quickly to our high-risk population. Some have severe, complicating medical issues, some are prone to accidents, and some end their lives by suicide.

We recently had a service for a man I'd worked with for years. He'd had a rough life with a history of traumas, no resources, and few acquaintances. He lived in a tiny space with a shared kitchen. More than anything, he wanted a cat but didn't think it would be fair to keep a pet in such confined conditions. He had diabetes but, most of the time, felt that it just wasn't worth the effort to take his medicine. And, ultimately, he died in his early fifties from his uncontrolled and uncared-for illness. I felt very sad...

Moments in clinic can be tense. Patients may present as intoxicated or in the midst of a crisis. With emotions out of control, they can have an outburst and frighten everyone around them. In these cases, clinic safety is foremost. All rooms are equipped with a panic alarm that alerts the front desk for instant backup. A security officer arrives, and the patient may be escorted to the emergency department for evaluation. "The biggest challenge," says Senior Clinic Manager Sunny Lovin, LICSW, "is when people don't want the care and the services we're offering and then we just have to figure out the best way to support them and keep everyone safe."

On a positive note, she goes on to say: "We consistently see patients who have been served by our clinic achieving really big recovery goals, like getting a job or finding permanent housing. People actually become well enough to move completely out of the system. They get off of Social Security Disability benefits then transition to getting most of their services from their primary physician and no longer need specialty care from our clinic. These are huge moments when you see this happen."

Lovin sees a bright future for the outpatient clinic with possible new space and the addition of even more services. Harborview Mental Health and Addiction Service fills an already great and ever-growing need in the community.

25

A Unique Program: The Clinic for Specialized Treatment in Early Psychosis

With a contribution by Christine E. Curry, MD

Schizophrenia, an illness that typically begins in young adulthood, may lead to a lifetime of disability. Researchers and clinicians find that effective treatment started in the earliest stages of the illness can reduce the ultimate severity of the outcomes of this debilitating disease.

The early years after psychotic symptoms first appear predict much of the eventual morbidity in schizophrenia and related disorders. The person can experience suicidality, violent behaviors, loss of function because of relapse, and subsequent hospitalizations. Substance misuse and social isolation often emerge. It is widely accepted that pharmacological and psychological interventions have ultimately improved outcomes if the patient is treated during this critical window of opportunity. Of particular promise are comprehensive first-episode services with teams that integrate and adapt the delivery of empirically based treatments to younger individuals and their families.

Ideally, treatment should begin even before the illness declares itself with its delusions, hallucinations, and loss of touch with reality. If patients in the prodromal stage began treatment before the onset of full-blown disease, the ultimate outcome could improve. Unfortunately, such early detection is not realistic but at least an intervention can start with an obvious first episode.

Early intervention, instituted as soon as possible after a first onset of psychosis, has proven possible, practical, and effective. For the past two decades, this phase-specific treatment has been used in the US and internationally, and specially created psychological, social, and medical management can be offered as supplement to standard care or provided through a special intervention team.

Harborview's Specialized Treatment in Early Psychosis (STEP) program, launched in 2019, is one of eight first-episode psychosis projects in Washington state. The team is staffed by providers from various disciplines: psychiatrists, social workers, nurses, and psychologists. Treatment begins with an assessment to understand the patient's background and current situation. Patient and team collaborate to set goals. Treatment includes some or all of several modalities with individual and group therapy; medication management; support to return to work or school; and education and assistance for family and friends.

STEP at Harborview is dedicated to intense and individualized care. Enrollment is kept to thirty participants at a time since the clinic strives to devote as much attention as possible to each patient. Clients are generally young, between the ages of sixteen and thirty. As with a healthy population of the same age, it can be challenging to encourage patients to follow suggestions from adults.

Providers address all aspects of the patient's needs. There is a full-time psychologist who offers behavior-focused psychotherapies such as individual resiliency training, a cognitive-behavioral treatment for issues resulting from psychosis. This therapy calls on strengths and concentrates on recovery goals, improving social function and overall well-being. STEP also offers cognitive behavioral therapy for psychotic symptoms whose aim is to reduce the stress of hearing voices and experiencing delusions including the intense fear of others. A case manager or a social worker offers family therapy to those involved in the patient's life as well as acts as clinic coordinator and program director. An employment and education specialist assists with exploring work and school options. The peer specialist, someone who has also experienced mental illness, serves as an important member of the team, as they give the patient a connection to an empathic person who truly understands their struggles and can engage in a way that others cannot.

Family support is primary. Families may see their relative's illness differently than the way the patient perceives it and may be frustrated as they try to figure out the best way to be helpful. Furthermore, they can be devastated by their own confusion and needs, so staff aid the family to understand their relation, to provide safety and support, and to navigate a complicated system.

Medical and psychiatric needs are addressed by the nurse and psychiatrist. The psychiatrist prescribes medications necessary to treat a psychotic disorder and makes changes in dose and regimen as needed. In addition to involvement with psychiatric care, the nurse attends to general issues for the client's comprehensive health. The nurse will make sure, for example, that the person engages with their primary provider because appointments and medical medicines among schizophrenia patients are often neglected. Nurses provide additional valuable services: They monitor the negative metabolic changes that often accompany antipsychotic medications, and they offer support and education to optimize health, including sexual health, a subject that often goes ignored.

Referrals to the STEP program primarily come from inpatient psychiatric units. The clinic maintains a website and advertises their services. Patients can self-refer, and families and other unrelated individuals can also encourage a patient to present to the clinic. The vision of the STEP clinic is to offer care and consultation to providers and patients in the community. It would benefit all if illness is caught and treated before hospitalization is the only option.

(26)

Dialectical Behavior Therapy

With contributions by Ann M. Allen, LICSW;
John T. Blatchford, LICSW, MHC; Lynn Elwood, LMHC;
Sunny Lovin, LICSW; and Carson Robinson, LICSW

Existing treatments for patients with borderline personality disorder (BPD) were mostly ineffective until the 1980s when psychologist Marsha Linehan developed a life-saving therapy. She recognized the need for a specialized approach for people plagued by chronic suicidality, impulsivity, and emotional and physical self-harming behaviors. Her approach could now offer hope to those experiencing intense and unmanageable negative emotions that damage relationships and prevent having a stable life.

Linehan found that a variation of cognitive behavioral therapy was effective in helping patients manage their dysregulated emotions. She devised dialectical behavior therapy (DBT) based on the notion that acceptance of holding two opposite perspectives is beneficial. Achieving balance and avoiding an all-or-nothing style fosters change for the better. Life can, by all indications, improve. The "dialectic" at the heart of DBT is acceptance and ultimate change.

By combining standard cognitive-behavioral techniques for emotional regulation with the concepts of tolerating distress and mindful awareness, DBT succeeds in improving the lives of patients with BPD. It is also effective for those bearing other diagnoses. DBT has proven valid for people recognized to have eating disorders as it helps patients establish coping mechanisms to reduce anxiety associated with food. DBT has been used to address drug and alcohol problems, post-traumatic stress, and mood disorders. Research has proven that DBT reduces the number of suicidal gestures, treatment dropouts, and frequent hospitalizations. Among patients with BPD, communication and interaction with others decidedly improve.

DBT relies on four modules: mindfulness, distress tolerance, emotion regulation, and interpersonal effectiveness. The treatment consists of individual therapy sessions and participation in DBT skills groups. Consultation meetings are routinely held for all of the program's specially trained therapists. The individual therapist encourages the patient to remain motivated and to practice the skills learned in group. They remain available to their clients for telephone coaching and support in moments of crisis. Clients redefine their identity as they incorporate the skills acquired in DBT into their daily lives.

Hospitalization is not a recognized treatment for patients with BPD and is, in fact, contraindicated except in emergency. DBT is designed to encourage independence, enhance coping skills, and avoid fostering dependence on hospital care. In past years patients could engage in a "high utilizer" program with planned, brief hospital stays that were not contingent on crisis. This was part of shaping a plan to ultimately reduce admissions and encourage managing challenges outside of the hospital.

Currently, three sections with ten patients each participate in Harborview's year-long program. During that time, they attend groups and meet with their individual therapist but, according to the treatment plan, that relationship must end at the completion of the year. Participants are then considered graduates. If they want to continue visits with their therapist and make further progress, they apply to the DBT-Accepting the Challenges of Employment and Self-Sufficiency (DBT-ACES), a program lasting for an additional year. The ultimate goal of DBT-ACES is to be able to forgo psychiatric disability and become self-sufficient by returning to the workforce.

Harborview's DBT program is one of thousands around the world but is unique in that it offers services in a community mental health setting. Participation is often limited by patient finances but, whereas many other programs are self-pay, Harborview accepts Medicaid and Medicare. Unfortunately, greater access results in a longer wait list and it could be a year or more until a there is an available place in the program.

Therapist Carson Robinson, LICSW, describes a few of the many successes he's seen:

> I'm now working with GK, a young woman who'd been calling the mobile crisis team on a weekly basis. She was causing all kinds of chaos in the system: She'd repeatedly present at the hospital; she was regularly and frequently calling the police and she'd threaten suicide each time she called the crisis line. She was also showing up at the clinic and telling anyone who would listen that she was going to kill herself. You can imagine what kind of pandemonium this caused. Her therapist was totally burned out. She's been in DBT now for the past six months and she's not had one contact with the mobile crisis team. It's fair to say that this woman's life has really turned around!

I have another client who spent years in residential programs. In the long run, these really didn't help much. Life has changed for her now that she's in DBT. She used to frequently lose control. She'd get arrested for domestic violence and when things would go bad for her, she'd threaten to stab herself. Six months into treatment she's now able to rein in her chaotic feelings, observe limits, and accept herself and others as they are.

Robinson describes the inevitability of failures over the years. Although not many in number, they are still distressing for the team. Some suicides do occur, and clients drop out of the program before they have reached maximum benefit. Clinicians make every effort possible to keep patients in treatment. When a client doesn't keep their appointment, providers try to explore the reasons and encourage them to continue care. It's not until they miss four sessions in a row that the relationship is terminated.

Lisa Lovejoy, a coordinator at the Housing and Recovery Through Peer Services (HARPS) program at Harborview Mental Health Services, publicly shares the story of her struggles with mental health issues so that others might be inspired to benefit from her experiences. Lovejoy's life was in turmoil: She lost her job and the custody of her children, she was overwhelmed with periods of depression and mania, and she had three hospitalizations and an overpowering sense of despair. Lovejoy was eventually directed to the DBT program which, she acknowledges, has rescued her from despondency. Now she can work, have meaningful relationships, and lives a purposeful and productive life.

Like Lovejoy's experience and the experience of thousands of others, DBT is indeed a life-saving treatment, giving the prospect of a useful and satisfying existence to those who had only been living in darkness.

(27)

Harborview Abuse & Trauma Center
Meeting the Community's Need

With a contribution by Laura Merchant, LICSW

Traumas of every kind afflict the adults and children of our community: sexual assault, child maltreatment and crime. Acute events are devastating, and their aftermath can be disastrous. Harborview Abuse & Trauma Center (HATC), established in 1973, provides for the support and treatment of trauma victims. Through the years, HATC has gone beyond treating only victims of rape to offering a wide range of services to all in need. As a certified Community Sexual Assault Program, Crime Victim Service Center, and partner in the King County Children's Justice Center, HATC is nationally recognized for its accomplishments.

Victims of sexual assault are provided with medical care and forensic evaluations. Those needing emergent treatment are seen by a Sexual Assault Nurse Examiner (SANE) at one of six King County medical center emergency departments. After evaluation, patients are offered a future appointment at HATC with a SANE provider and medical social worker. These optional visits are available for those who have additional questions, who would benefit from a second examination, or have continued distress. During this appointment, needs are evaluated, and the victim is provided with information, advocacy, support, and brief psychological help. The team also offers the option for longer-term counseling. Child victims are assessed and treated by medical providers trained in caring for abused children. Initial forensic medical SANE exams are covered through Washington State Crime Victim's Compensation; initial counseling appointments are offered at no charge.

HATC offers many free services that provide information, referrals, crisis management, and support including advocacy for medical and legal needs. Ongoing therapy is available and is financed by various resources. One option is several brief sessions focusing on psychoeducation and strengthening resiliency. Other treatments provide trauma-specific interventions such as Cognitive Processing Therapy, Prolonged Exposure, Common Elements Treatment Approach for Adults, and Trauma-Focused Cognitive Behavioral Therapy for children. HATC also offers trauma-focused parenting interventions as well as addressing depressive and anxiety-related symptoms resulting from traumatic experiences.

HATC has a long history of being part of a coordinated community response to victims in need. It operates a Foster Care Assessment Program funded by Washington State's Department of Children, Youth, and Families. This program assists social workers with consultation aimed at improving child and youth well-being and aids with finding permanent placement for victims. HATC administers statewide learning collaboratives to mental health organizations on evidence-based trauma therapies with in-person training and monthly group case consultation by telephone. HATC also arranges SANE training throughout the state. As part of the

King County Children's Justice Center, HATC works closely with its community partners. HATC is committed to preventing abuse by active involvement in statewide and community initiatives and programs to end interpersonal violence.

HATC has always been on the cutting edge of trauma services. Its recently retired director Lucy Berliner, a widely respected expert, continues to provide consultation and guidance, and the program's current director, Laura Merchant, maintains the tradition of responding to victims' needs. HATC is—and will remain—a powerful addition to the arsenal of services provided at Harborview.

(28)

Research at Harborview

With contributions by David Avery, MD; Lydia Chwastiak, MD, MPH; Sarah Kopelovich, PhD; Maria Monroe-DeVita, PhD; Sunila Nair, MBBS, PhD; John Neumaier, MD, PhD; Richard K. Ries, MD; Mark Snowden, MD, MPH; and Douglas Zatzick, MD

The University of Washington is recognized as an academic institution whose research programs span its six hospitals. Harborview's research is active and ongoing with funding provided by national and private sources. Put simply, researchers in the Department of Psychiatry and Behavioral Sciences seek basic understanding of the brain and behaviors and, using the information gathered, they aim to make discoveries that will lead to better treatments for mental illness, substance use disorders, and problems caused by chronic pain.

To document all the projects currently ongoing at Harborview would require a heavy textbook (print, not an eBook) so only a few are highlighted to give an idea of the general scope of current research activities. Some conduct projects based on clinical information while others, like Dr. John Neumaier, work in a laboratory staffed by a dozen or more graduate students, post-doctoral fellows, technicians, undergraduates, and a laboratory manager.

DAVID AVERY, MD

Recruited upon completion of his National Institute of Mental Health Post-Doctoral Fellowship at the University of Copenhagen's Psychochemistry Institute, David Avery joined the faculty at the University of Washington's Harborview Medical Center in 1980. David Dunner, Chief of Psychiatry, invited Avery to enhance the hospital's research activities as well as to contribute his clinical skills. Avery remained with the Department of Psychiatry until 2012, serving as clinician and making important and internationally recognized scientific contributions.

Starting in 1985, Avery was an early investigator in the fields of winter depression, circadian rhythms and bright light therapy. He found that light treatment administered in the morning was effective in treating the depression that results from winter's dim ambient light. Taking his work one step further, he learned that depression could lift with early morning exposure to a dawn-light simulating device. Noting that depressed patients sometimes sleep excessively, he found that gradually increasing illumination in the bedroom prior to awakening was an effective treatment. Of interest, he also identified that abnormal circadian rhythms compounding depression could be shifted toward a normal spectrum with carefully timed exposure to bright light.

In the 1990's Avery's attention turned to transcranial magnetic stimulation (TMS), a relatively new treatment for depression. This noninvasive procedure involves delivering repetitive magnetic pulses that target areas of the brain identified as associated with depressive symptoms by means of a coil placed on the scalp. The first device was introduced in 1985 for treating patients who showed no improvement with medication or psychotherapy. Funded by the National Institute of Mental Health, Avery participated in a large, multi-site study demonstrating TMS's effectiveness, the results of which led to the Food and Drug Administration's approval of this treatment in 2008.

Over the course of his career, Avery has co-authored many articles and book chapters, been an invited presenter for national and international meetings, served as Principal Investigator for a dozen grants and serves as referee for multiple academic journals. Harborview and the University of Washington are proud to have had this researcher and clinician on its faculty for three decades.

LYDIA CHWASTIAK, MD, MPH

Over the past decade, Chwastiak has combined her clinical and research interests. She cares for patients with various serious mental illnesses and her research focuses on the intersection of chronic medical illness with psychiatric conditions. For example, she has examined the cardiovascular risk factors and healthcare costs among veterans with mental illness. Among her recent projects is the development of a community mental health center-based team approach to treating poorly controlled type 2 diabetes among outpatients with schizophrenia.

DAVID DUNNER, MD

David Dunner, born in Brooklyn, NY in 1940, was the initial force introducing research to Harborview. Before completing residency in 1969, he began his studies of bipolar disorder starting with an unpublished study of the effect of ECT in the treatment of acute mania. He was one of the first to use the experimental drug, lithium carbonate which he obtained by asking the pharmacy to prepare capsules from their stock bottles of the chemical. Dunner worked for two years from 1969 – 71 at the National Institute of Mental Health (NIMH) where he joined a group studying the biochemistry of manic-depressive illness. One accomplishment of that era was an assay for catechol-O-methyltransferase (COMT) in the blood of patients with depression and schizophrenia co-authored with Nobel Prize winner, Julius Axelrod and published in *Science.*

Two of Dunner's achievements were the identification of Bipolar II and of rapid cycling, diagnoses considered invaluable today. In addition, his early studies focused on the genetics of bipolar disorder, a subject that didn't arouse much scientific enthusiasm because the general consensus was that this illness wasn't of a biologic etiology but mainly caused by psychosocial factors.

After leaving NIMH Dunner continued his research on bipolar disorder working with Ronald Fieve at Columbia University's Lithium Clinic in New York. At the time, lithium was negatively viewed in the United States because it had caused death when used as a sodium substitute in cardiac patients. Fieve was instrumental in gaining greater acceptance of this valuable drug.

In 1979, Dunner relocated to the University of Washington as Chief of Psychiatry at Harborview. Here he developed a large program of clinical trials. Within five years of arrival, organized 26 ongoing studies and, with the benefit of money from grants, was able to fund young researchers at the University. In the mid-1980's he created The Center for Anxiety and Depression staffed by faculty experts. In addition, he developed a consulting service for local clinicians and introduced structured assessments of patients as a research tool. Dunner achieved recognition as Seattle's clinical expert in bipolar disorder and treatment resistant depression.

Dunner's scope of research was broad. He ran trials of antidepressants, anxiolytics and neuroleptics, one of which—Risperidone—is an accepted treatment today. Dunner's research expanded into psychotherapy as well. For example, he developed studies comparing the effectiveness of CBT and fluoxetine in dysthymia.

David Dunner's career has spanned decades and he currently continues with research studies and in private practice. He has authored or collaborated on 350 published papers, 10 books, served as president of multiple scientific societies and received numerous awards. Harborview and the Department of Psychiatry take pride in having had such an eminent scientist and clinician on staff.

SARAH KOPELOVICH, PHD

Kopelovich, a psychologist who has additional training in forensics, focuses her research on schizophrenic spectrum disorders and first episode psychosis. Her aim is to implement interventions for addressing this population's psychosocial and psychotherapeutic needs. Her work is evidence-based, and her goal is to make the results of her research accessible to providers and patients.

One of Kopelovich's projects is to increase availability of cognitive behavioral therapy (CBT) for psychosis in outpatient, inpatient, and forensic settings; She brings her work to the local community and to providers across the country. To that end, she developed and directs the first Project ECHO (Extension for Community Healthcare Outcomes) clinic that focuses on schizophrenia treatment. The ECHO project is a nationally recognized model for connecting expert specialist teams at an academic 'hub' with primary care clinicians in local communities by means of teleconferencing technology. Since 2015, she has directed the northwest CBT for Psychosis Provider Network, the only such professional development system in North America. In another project described in her most recent publication that appeared in 2019, she writes about "stepped care" as a system of delivering, implementing, and monitoring mental health treatment. Here, the most effective yet least resource-intensive treatment is delivered first and is only "stepped up" to more comprehensive services when needed.

MARIA MONROE-DEVITA, PHD

Monroe-DeVita's research interests are devoted to helping individuals with serious mental illness. She aims at developing and testing novel approaches to better serve people with these conditions and has been making her academic contributions as a part of the Harborview community for the past decade and a half.

A focus of Monroe-DeVita's work has been the Assertive Community Treatment (ACT) model. In this system, first introduced in 1980, researchers challenged standard practices in psychiatry by concluding that instruction to prepare patients for community living after hospital discharge was ineffective. They proposed that providing training and support within the community after leaving hospitalization was more useful. The principles of *assessment, training, and support* became the basis of the ACT model, which relies on *assertive outreach* to engage clients. The ACT team offers help with managing illness, finances, housing, and anything else necessary to assist in adjustment to community life.

As a researcher, Monroe-DeVita has served as Principal Investigator for projects developing, implementing, and assessing ten new ACT teams within the Washington state Division of Behavioral Health and Recovery. Her work also includes creating pilot programs for Illness Management and Recovery, a program that helps patients learn how to handle their illness in collaboration with treatment providers and integrated dual disorder treatment, a practice that improves the quality of life for people with co-occurring severe mental illness and substance use disorders by combined chemical dependency and mental health services.

SUNILA NAIR, MBBS, PHD

Relapse is a critical and unsolved problem in the treatment of addiction. Despite decades of effort, the neuronal mechanisms that drive relapse are incompletely understood. Nair investigates the functional neural circuitry that underlies relapse to drugs of abuse. She considers the role of non-drug reinforcers, substances that are meant to give sufficient satisfaction when offered in place of the craved drug. Presenting these alternatives have been found to provide a potential method for treating substance use disorders.

Nair works with various complex behavior models combining pharmacology with synthetically engineered tools as she seeks to define what is involved in relapse. Currently, she's focused on the role of a particular area of the brain, the lateral habenula, in her exploration of the causes of relapse.

JOHN F. NEUMAIER, MD, PHD

Neumaier is an attending psychiatrist at Harborview and is head of the Division of Psychiatric Neurosciences in the Department of Psychiatry and Behavioral Sciences at the University of Washington. He is also associate director of the UW Alcohol & Drug Abuse Institute.

Dr. Neumaier's clinical interests include treatment resistant mood and psychotic disorders. His research focuses on studying complex emotional behaviors involving addiction, learning, motivation, and stress. By examining responses in rodent models using molecular, pharmacological, and behavioral strategies, Neumaier can assess the reactions he sees and aims to look at what can be done to alter them.

Neumaier's laboratory focuses on investigating the interface of pharmacology, molecular neuroscience, and behavior. They look at several parameters including RNA regulation, protein translation, cellular plasticity, and neural circuit level analysis of complex behaviors relating to stress and addiction models. In addition to using rat and mouse behavioral models, they also rely on in-vitro cultures of cell lines and primary neurons to study how signals are transmitted inside the cell. These signals ultimately produce observable behaviors that might be relevant to those seen in humans.

A laboratory such as Neumeier's must be funded by grants, mostly from the National Institute of Health. It can take up to five years for a research project to fully mature with observable results, so Neumaier must be constantly publishing along the way on what he finds. The advantage of publications is that grant reviewers reading the papers are kept informed of the progress his laboratory has made and of the new methods they've developed.

Neumaier's laboratory was hit hard by the 2019 radiation contamination. Unable to work safely in his usual and comfortable space, his laboratory is now spread over several UW facilities and will ultimately be relocated to the VA.

RICHARD K. RIES, MD.

Ries is another senior researcher whose credentials include being the director of Outpatient Psychiatry, Dual Disorder Programs, the Chemical Dependency Project at Harborview, and the Division of Addictions for the Department of Psychiatry.

Reis' research focuses on the field of addictions. He obtained National Institute of Drug Abuse-sponsored clinical research grants in 1989 and 1997 to evaluate treatment outcome in dual disorders. He has since gone on to work on the project module, Preventing Addiction-Related Suicide (PARS).

Reis recognized that persons addicted to alcohol and drugs are at 5–10 times higher risk for suicide as compared to the general population. To address the need for improved suicide prevention strategies in this population, he developed PARS. In the pilot study, patients demonstrated that they knew more about suicide prevention then they were aware of before treatment. At one month after treatment, they were better able to cope with suicidal impulses. Clinic staff also commended PARS and decided that it could be used in their standard clinical practice.

The PARS pilot has expanded to a NIDA/NIMH funded intervention study with the collaboration of Kathryn Comtois, PhD. Nine hundred patients are enrolled in this unique examination of suicide prevention in a high-risk population. Because of success, PARS is now being developed for use with Alaska Native/American Indians and veterans. Versions are currently being created for treating the emotional challenges faced by first responders and individuals who are dependent on opioids.

PETER ROY-BYRNE, MD

After training at the University of California Los Angeles' Neuropsychiatric Hospital and the National Institutes of Health Clinical Center, Peter Roy-Byrne became the Department of Psychiatry and Behavioral Science's Vice Chair and Chief of Psychiatry at the Harborview Medical Center in 1992. He remained in this position as clinical expert and National Institute of Mental Health-funded researcher focusing on the evaluation and treatment of complex mood and anxiety disorders until 2011.

While at Harborview, Roy-Byrne earned recognition for directing the results of his scientific investigation for the benefit of clinical practice. In early years as a researcher, he focused on the neurobiology of mood and anxiety disorders and had a special interest in the role played by benzodiazepine receptors in these conditions.

Roy-Byrne identified the need for primary care providers to have understanding and skill to treat mood disorders. He served as Chair of participating Principal Investigators of the Collaborative Care for Anxiety and Panic (CCAP) project that involved the University of Washington, University of California Los Angeles, University of California San Diego and the Rand Corporation. He directed his research efforts to introduce evidence-based treatments for patients suffering from anxiety to the primary care setting. The study conclusively demonstrated that a combination treatment with medication and cognitive behavioral therapy by trained primary care providers was more effective than care-as-usual in terms of cost and positive clinical results.

Upon completion of CCAP, Roy-Byrne continued to chair a committee of Principal Investigators at the same sites plus and additional clinical location at the University of Arkansas. The CCAP model was expanded to Coordinated Anxiety Learning and Management (CALM) to include all four anxiety disorders—panic, posttraumatic stress, generalized anxiety and social anxiety disorders. The study examined ways in which primary care clinicians could improve the strategies for treatment of anxiety disorders that were already in use. Results demonstrated that those patients who had received CALM's interventions had fewer symptoms of anxiety than those receiving standard treatment.

Roy-Byrne always had the Harborview mission in mind as he participated in the Center for Healthcare Improvement for Addictions, Mental Illness and Medically Vulnerable Populations as a Center of Emphasis established in 2006.

Although Roy-Byrne left Harborview to devote his time to his group psychiatric practice, he continues to make significant contributions to his chosen field. He is Editor-in-Chief of *New England Journal of Medicine Journal Watch Psychiatry* and is Co-Editor-in-Chief of *UpToDate Psychiatry* and adds to the scientific literature that already lists his 400 publications.

Peter Roy-Byrne will always be remembered for the legacy he has left as a Harborview clinician and researcher.

MARK SNOWDEN, MD, MPH

Chief of Service Mark Snowden's clinical work involves the care of elder patients. His research explores the delivery of evidence-based mental health services to older adults.

Depression in this population is a serious and widespread condition that impacts social, emotional and physical well-being. If depressive symptoms can be treated, life is less overwhelming and more satisfying. In the 1990's the University of Washington Health Promotion Research Center was asked to address this condition and so the Program to Encourage Active, Rewarding Lives (PEARLS) was born. Snowden, a dissemination and implementation researcher, collaborated to create a program that has since grown to improve the lives of elders throughout the country.

Local aging service providers partner with the University to implement PEARLS. Care is offered to elders in need of relief from depression who are frail and often home bound. Participants needn't come to a hospital or clinic: treatment can be delivered in the comfort of their own home or in an accessible community setting. PEARLS' facilitators work as a team to provide a brief, home-based course. Seniors – even those with chronic medical conditions—learn tools to effectively tackle overwhelming obstacles in their lives. As a result, distressing symptoms are relieved, and outlook and function improve. This structured intervention is delivered in 6 to 8 one-hour visits over 5 months.

PEARLS is successful! In 2004, Paul Ciechanowski, MD, MPH, a University of Washington psychiatrist, documented its effectiveness in a study published in the *Journal of the American Medical Association*. Since then, further reports have appeared in the scientific literature showing that this evidence-based program can dramatically reduce depression and improve quality of life.

Snowden's work in this area has continued since its introduction. He received a 2007-2010 R-18 translational research grant that allowed his group to explore implementation of PEARLS with King County's Aging and Disability Services (ADS), the original partner in the PEARLS effectiveness trial. ADS was struggling with the challenges of carrying out the project in actual practice. Snowden's group sought to increase the program's area of delivery. In partnership with ADS, their efforts changed the Washington State Medicaid Waiver policy so that PEARLS could be funded by state Medicaid dollars for eligible residents. Another accomplishment was the passing of a King County levy to include funding for underserved minorities and veterans. In recognition of their achievements, the group received the American Public Health Association's Aging and Public Health Section 2011 Archstone Award for Excellence in Program Innovation.

Snowden and colleagues now offer PEARLS trainings to groups across the country and provide monthly technical assistance by teleconference. As a result, there are now over 50 PEARLS programs in 20 states.

Snowden's current research explores employing PEARLS as a means to decrease inequities in health care by collaborating with community-based organizations serving patients of color and for those with low income. The primary language of many in the community is not English; PEARLS has been modified so all can experience its benefits.

The work of Mark Snowden, clinician, administrator and researcher, has made an enduring contribution to the well-being of our elder population.

DOUGLAS ZATZICK, MD

Zatzick is professor in the Department of Psychiatry & Behavioral Sciences. His research focus has been the investigation of trauma and the effects it has on those who have experienced disaster. Over the past two decades he's developed a public health approach to trauma as seen in acute care medical settings. His clinical trials have targeted post-traumatic stress disorder and related co-morbid conditions such as depression, suicidal ideation, and alcohol and drug use problems among injured youth and adults.

Currently, Zatzick is the Principal Investigator of an NIH Healthcare Systems Research Collaboratory/NIMH-sponsored study. This investigation examines the effectiveness of screening and treatment of PTSD and co-morbid conditions in twenty-five level I trauma center sites across the nation.

Bibliography

BEGINNINGS: THE HISTORY OF HARBORVIEW MEDICAL CENTER

A Seattle Hospital for Everyone. (n.d.). Retrieved December 10, 2019, from https://www.uwmedicine.org/locations/harborview-medical-center. A Seattle Hospital for Everyone. Accessed December 10, 2019

Adaptive reuse potential of Harborview Hall. (n.d.). Retrieved December 13, 2019, from https://historicseattle.org/adaptive-reuse-potential-of-harborview-hall/

Art Deco. (n.d.). Retrieved December 12, 2019, from https://www.britannica.com/art/Art-Deco.

Bulger, E., Kastl, J., & Maier, R. (2017). The history of Harborview Medical Center and the Washington State Trauma System. *Trauma Surg Acute Care Open.*, *2*(1). https://doi.org/10.1136/tsaco-2017-000091

Ensign, J. (2017, June 22). The Hospital on Profanity Hill—A History of Harborview Hospital (Seattle) By Josephine Ensign. . Retrieved December 12, 2019, from https://www.historylink.org/File/20393. The Hospital on Profanity Hill—A History of Harborview Hospital (Seattle) By Josephine Ensign. Posted 6/22/2017.

Gonzalez, S. (2017, March 9). A History of Harborview Medical Center. Retrieved December 10, 2017, from https://blogs.uw.edu/gonzalsa/2017/03/09/a-history-on-harborview-medical-center/

Harborview Medical Center. (n.d.). Retrieved December 9, 2019, from https://en.wikipedia.org/wiki/Harborview_Medical_Center.

Harborview Medical Center Ninth and Jefferson Building. (n.d.-a). Retrieved December 13, 2019, from https://www.turnerconstruction.com/experience/project/45F/harborview-medical-center-ninth-jefferson-building

Harborview Medical Center Ninth and Jefferson Building. (n.d.-b). Retrieved December 13, 2019, from https://www.mka.com/projects/featured/harborview-medical-center-9th-and-jefferson

Harborview Medical Center's 257 million expansion almost complete. (n.d.). Retrieved December 13, 2019, from https://www.seattletimes.com/seattle-news/harborview-medical-centers-257-million-expansion-almost-complete/

Harborview Research and Training. (n.d.). Retrieved December 13, 2019, from http://www.wjcengineers.com/harborviewresearchandtraining

Historic preservation projects. (n.d.). Retrieved December 13, 2019, from https://www.kingcounty.gov/services/home-property/historic-preservation/projects/harborview-hall.aspx. Accessed December 20, 2019

King County Hospital. Harborview to be one of finest in United States. (1931, February 22). *The Seattle Sunday Times*, p. 6.

Obituary. Norm Maleng. (n.d.). Retrieved December 13, 2019, from https://www.legacy.com/obituaries/seattletimes/obituary.aspx?n=norm-maleng&pid=88447821

Preserving Harborview Hall. (n.d.). Retrieved December 13, 2019, from http://www.preservewa.org/most_endangered/harborview-hall/

Radiation-incident-in-research-facility-on-Harborview-campus. . (n.d.). Retrieved December 12, 2019, from https://www.doh.wa.gov/Newsroom/Articles/ID/356/Radiation-incident-in-research-facility-on-Harborview-campus.

Sheffield, J., Young, A., Goldstein, E., & Logerfo, J. (2016). The public hospital mission at Seattle's Harborview Medical Center: high-quality care for the underserved and excellence in medical education. *Acad Med.* , *81*(10), 886–890. https://doi.org/10.1097/01.ACM.0000238118.63470.5b

PSYCHIATRY'S HISTORY AT HARBORVIEW

Commissioners Yield After Judge Criticizes Hospital. (1931, April 7) *The Seattle Daily Times*, Second Main News Section.

Drake, RE, Green, AI, Mueser, KT, & Goldman, HH. (2003). The history of community mental health treatment and rehabilitation for persons with severe mental illness. *Community Ment Health J.* , 39(5), 427–440. https://doi.org/10.1023/a:1025860919277

Drake, R., & Latimer, E. (2012). Lessons learned in developing community mental health care in North America. *World Psychiatry.* , 11(1), 47–51. https://doi.org/10.1016/j.wpsyc.2012.01.007.

Hadley, J. (2002, July 9). Pat Steel, widely respected veteran county employee, dies at 57. Retrieved February 3, 2020, from https://www.seattlepi.com/news/article/Pat-Steel-widely-respected-veteran-county-1090960.php

Thomas, C. (2013, November 22). 50 Years after the Community Mental Health Act, The Best Reporting on Mental Health Care Today. Retrieved January 2, 2020, from https://psmag.com/social-justice/50-years-community-mental-health-act-best-reporting-mental-health-care-today-70353.

Tomito, S. (2018, September 6). Remembering ACRS' earliest years and celebrating its progress. Retrieved January 2, 2020, from https://iexaminer.org/remembering-acrs-earliest-years-and-celebrating-its-progress/

MARK SNOWDEN, MD, MPH: CHIEF OF SERVICE

Mark Snowden, MD, MPH. (n.d.). Retrieved January 3, 2020, from https://medicine.uw.edu/faculty/clinical-practice/university-washington-physicians.

Designated Crisis Responders. (n.d.). Retrieved April 8, 2020, from https://www.hca.wa.gov/billers-providers-partners/ behavioral-health-recovery/designated-crisis-responders-dcr

Saklayen, M. (2018). The Global Epidemic of Metabolic Syndrome. *Current Hypertension Reports, 20*(2), 1–8. https://doi.org/10.1007/s11906-018-0812-z

THE PSYCHIATRY EMERGENCY SERVICE
Workplace Violence in Healthcare. (n.d.). Retrieved February 3, 2020, from https://www.osha.gov/Publications/OSHA3826.pdf.

Designated Crisis Responders. (n.d.). Retrieved December 25, 2019, from https://www.hca.wa.gov/billers-providers-partners/ behavioral-health-recovery/designated-crisis-responders-dcr.

Hooker, E., Mallow, P., & Oglesby, M. (2019). Characteristics and Trends of Emergency Department Visits in the United States (2010-2014). *J Emerg Med, 56*(3), 344–351. https://doi.org/10.1016/j.jemermed.2018.12.025

Leder, L., & Chatmon, B. (2019). Treatment and Outcomes in Adult Designated Psychiatric Emergency Service Units. *Crit Care Nurs Clin North Am.* , *31*(2), 225–236. https://doi.org/10.1016/j.cnc.2019.02.008.Epub2019

Levin-Epstein, M. (2015, November 18). Psych Units in the ED: Trend, Solution, or Neither? Retrieved February 1, 2020, from https://epmonthly.com/article/ psych-units-in-the-ed-trend-solution-or-neither/

Midwicket, M. (2018). Factors Associated with Emergency Department Use by Patients with and Without Mental Health Diagnoses. *JAMA Network Open* , *1*(6), 1–7. https://doi.org/10.1001/jamanetworkopen.2018.3528

Nitkin, K. (2018, October 19). The Changing Dynamics of Emergency Care. Retrieved February 4, 2020, from https://www.hopkinsmedicine.org/news/articles/the-changing-dynamics-of-emergency-psychiatric-care

Nordstrom, K., Berlin, J., Nash, S., Shah, S., Schmeltzer, N., & Worley, L. (2019). Boarding of Mentally Ill Patients in Emergency Departments: American Psychiatric Association Resource Document. *West J Emerg Med.* , *20*(5), 690–695. https://doi.org/10.5811/westjem.2019.6.42422

Parker-Pope, T. (2010, February 18). 7 Secrets of the Emergency Room. Retrieved February 5, 2020, from https://well.blogs.nytimes.com/2010/02/18/7-secrets-of-the-emergency-room/

Should Mental Illness Be Treated in the ER? (n.d.). Retrieved February 5, 2020, from https://genesight.com/should-mental-illness-be-treated-in-the-er

The Function and Characteristics of Psychiatric Emergency Service. (n.d.). Retrieved February 5, 2020, from https://pitjournal.unc.edu/content/function-and-characteristics-psychiatric-emergency-service

Zeller, S., Calma, N., & Stone, A. (2014). Effects of a dedicated regional psychiatric emergency service on boarding of psychiatric patients in area emergency departments. *Est J Emerg Med.*, *15*(1), 1–6. https://doi.org/10.5811/westjem.2013.6.17848

THE PSYCHIATRIC INTENSIVE CARE UNIT
Inpatient Psychiatric Capacity in Washington State: Assessing Future Needs. (n.d.). Retrieved December 17, 2019, from https://www.wsipp.wa.gov/ReportFile/1092/Wsipp_Inpatient-Psychiatric-Capacity-in-Washington-State-Assessing-Future-Needs-and-Impacts-Part-One_Full-Report.pdf

Mental Health by the Numbers. (n.d.). Retrieved December 17, 2019, from https://www.nami.org/learn-more/mental-health-by-the-numbers.

Should Healthcare Workers Press Charges Against Violent Patients. (2018, November 16). Retrieved December 4, 2019, from https://www.washingtonpost.com/national/health-science/should-health-care-workers-press-charges-against-violent-patients

THERAPIES: OT/PT/RT
Patterson, C. (2008). A Short History of Occupational Therapy. In *Occupational Therapy and Mental Health* (pp. 3–16). Philadelphia, Pennsylvania: Churchill Livingstone/Elsevier.

PHARMACY

Canales, P., Dorson, P., & Crismon, M. (2001). Outcomes assessment of clinical pharmacy services in a psychiatric inpatient setting. *Am J Health Syst Pharm.*, 58(14), 1309–1316. https://doi.org/10.1093/ajhp/58.14.1309

Kantorovich, A. (2016, August 24). Gabapentin for Alcohol Use Disorder: A Promising Outlook. Retrieved June 14, 2020, from https://www.pharmacytimes.com/contributor/alexander-kantorovich-pharmd-bcps/2016/08/gabapentin-for-alcohol-use-disorder-a-promising-outlook

PEER BRIDGERS

Peer Bridgers and Peer Support Pilot . (n.d.). Retrieved March 3, 2020, from https://www.kingcounty.gov/~/media/depts/community-human-services/MIDD/initiatives/RR-11.ashx?la=en

What is the Peer Bridger Model of Peer Support. (n.d.). Retrieved March 2, 2020, from https://smiadviser.org/knowledge_post/what-is-the-peer-bridger-model-of-peer-support.

CONSULT-LIAISON PSYCHIATRY

Ostermeyer, B. (2017). Overview of Consultation-Liaison Psychiatry. *Psychiatric Annals*, 47(4), 168–169. https://doi.org/10.3928/00485713-20170308-01

Medical Consultation for Psychiatry

Thompson, R. (2019, February 15). Amazing Work We Get to Do. Retrieved March 26, 2020, from https://www.the-hospitalist.org/hospitalist/article/194620/leadership-training/amazing-work-we-get-do.

THE LAW AND PSYCHIATRY
Testa, M., & West, S.G. (2010). Civil commitment in the United States. *Psychiatry (Edgmont (Pa. : Township)), 7 10*, 30-40.

ADDRESSING CHEMICAL DEPENDENCY
Agerwala, S. (2012). Integrating Screening, Brief Intervention, and Referral to Treatment (SBIRT) into Clinical Practice Settings: A Brief Review. *J Psychoactive Drugs, 44*(4), 307–317. https://doi.org/10.1080/02791072.2012.720169.

Hicks, M. (n.d.). A Step into Integrated Care. Retrieved January 6, 2020, from https://cabhp.asu.edu/sites/default/files/session-4-pdf-presentation-hicks.pdf

Mental Health and Addiction Services at Harborview. (n.d.). Retrieved March 19, 2020, from https://www.uwmedicine.org/locations/addictions-program-harborview

Screening, brief intervention, and referral to treatment (SBIRT). (n.d.). Retrieved March 19, 2020, from https://www.hca.wa.gov/billers-providers-partners/behavioral-health-recovery/screening-brief-intervention-and-referral

Study shows power of supportive care for alcohol addiction. (n.d.). Retrieved January 2, 2020, from https://newsroom.uw.edu/postscript/study-shows-power-supportive-care-alcohol-addiction

PSYCHIATRISTS SHARE THEIR SKILLS

Behavioral Health Integration Program. (n.d.). Retrieved March 30, 2020, from https://aims.uw.edu/behavioral-health-integration-program-bhip

Boynton, L., Bentley, J., Jackson, J., & Gibbs, T. (2010). The Role of Stigma and State in the Mental Health of Somalis. *Journal of Psychiatric Practice, 16,* 265–268. https://doi.org/10.1097/01.pra.0000386914.85182.78

Karfatian, E. (2019). Lessons Learned in Prison and Jail-Based Telepsychiatry. *Curr Psychiatry Rep, 21*(3), 1–7. https://doi.org/10.1007/s11920-019-1004-5

Mental Health and Illness in Vietnamese Refugees. (n.d.). Retrieved March 3, 2020, from https://ethnomed.org/resource/mental-health-and-illness-in-vietnamese-refugees/

Partnership Access Line for Moms. (n.d.). Retrieved March 26, 2020, from https://providerresource.uwmedicine.org/videos/partnership-access-line-pal-for-moms1

What is Telepsychiatry. (n.d.). Retrieved March 26, 2020, from https://www.psychiatry.org/patients-families/what-is-telepsychiatry

ELECTROCONVULSIVE THERAPY

What is Electroconvulsive Therapy? (n.d.). Retrieved March 5, 2020, from https://www.psychiatry.org/patients-families/ect

GERIATRIC PSYCHIATRY

2019. Alzheimer's Disease. Facts and Figures. (n.d.). Retrieved March 29, 2020, from https://www.alz.org/media/documents/alzheimers-facts-and-figures-2019-r.pdf

SUICIDE: PREVENTION AND RECOVERY

About Suicide. (n.d.). Retrieved April 3, 2020, from https://www.americashealthrankings.org/explore/annual/measure/Suicide/state/WA

Coping with a client's suicide. (n.d.). Retrieved April 3, 2020, from https://www.apa.org/gradpsych/2008/11/suicide

Gillihan, S. (2018, September 16). What happens when you mention suicide in therapy. Retrieved April 3, 2020, from https://www.psychologytoday.com/us/blog/think-act-be/201809/what-happens-when-you-mention-suicide-in-therapy

Hawgood, J. (n.d.). Working with suicidal clients: Impacts on psychologists and the need for self-care. Retrieved April 21, 2020, from https://www.psychology.org.au/inpsych/2015/february/hawgood/

Jobes, D., Wong, S., Conrad, A., Drozd, J., & Neal-Walden, T. (2005). The collaborative assessment and management of suicidality versus treatment as usual: a retrospective study with suicidal outpatients. *Suicide & Life-Threatening Behavior, 35*(5), 483–497. https://doi.org/10.1521/suli.2005.35.5.483.

Karakurt, G., Anderson, A., Badford, A., Dial, S., & Korkow, H. (2014). Strategies for Managing Difficult Clinical Situations in Between Sessions. *The American Journal of Family Therapy, 42*(5), 413–425. https://doi.org/10.1080/01926187.2014.909657

Luxton, D., June, J., & Comtois, K. (2013). Can Post-Discharge Follow-Up Contacts Prevent Suicide and Suicidal Behavior? *Crisis, 34*(1), 32–41. https://doi.org/10.1027/0227-5910/a000158.

Suicide Statistics. (n.d.). Retrieved April 3, 2020, from https://afsp.org/suicide-statistics/

Zoler, L. (2018, May 4). Suicide prevention starts with the patient's narrative. Retrieved April 6, 2020, from https://www.mdedge.com/psychiatry/article/164933/depression/suicide-prevention-starts-patients-narrative

DIALECTICAL BEHAVIOR THERAPY

A Lifeline to Mental Health. (n.d.). Retrieved May 23, 2020, from https://www.washington.edu/boundless/harborview-mental-health/

Comtois, K., Kerbrat, A., Atkins, D., Harned, M., & Elwood, L. (2010, November 1). Recovery From Disability for Individuals With Borderline Personality Disorder: A Feasibility Trial of DBT-ACES. Retrieved April 3, 2020, from https://ps.psychiatryonline.org/doi/full/10.1176/ps.2010.61.11.1106?url_ver=Z39.88-2003&rfr_id=ori:rid:crossref.org&rfr_dat=cr_pub%3dpubmed

Dialectical Behavior Therapy. (n.d.). Retrieved April 3, 2020, from https://www.psychologytoday.com/us/therapy-types/dialectical-behavior-therapy

SPECIALIZED TREATMENT IN EARLY PSYCHOSIS

Meyer, P., Gottlieb, J., Penn, D., Mueser, K., & Gingerich, S. (n.d.). Individual Resiliency Training: An Early Intervention Approach to Enhance Well-Being in People with First Break Psychosis. Retrieved April 4, 2020, from http://www.navigate-consultants.org/wp-content/uploads/2017/05/Meyer-2015.pdf

Srihari, V., Kucukgoncu, S., Phutane, V., Breitborde, N., Pollard, J., & Ozkan, B. (2015). First-Episode Services for Psychotic Disorders in the U.S. Public Sector: A Pragmatic Randomized Controlled Trial. *Psychiatric Services (Washington, D.C.), 66*(7), 705–712. https://doi.org/10.1176/appi.ps.201400236

HARBORVIEW ABUSE & TRAUMA CENTER

Descriptions of more Harborview Abuse & Trauma Center services are available at www.uwhatc.org

More information can be found at https://depts.washington.edu/hcsats/FCAP/

Information on sexual assault medical services, and advocacy and counseling services, can be found at http://depts.washington.edu//hcsats/ch/index.html

RESEARCH

Avery, D. H., Claypoole, K., Robinson, L., Neumaier, J. F., Dunner, D. L., Scheele, L., Wilson, L., & Roy-Byrne, P. (1999). Repetitive Transcranial Magnetic Stimulation in the Treatment of Medication-Resistant Depression: Preliminary Data. *The Journal of Nervous & Mental Disease, 187*(2), 114–117. https://doi.org/10.1097/00005053-199902000-0000

Avery, D. H., Khan, A., Dager, S. R., Cohen, S., Cox, G. B., & Dunner, D. L. (1991). Morning or evening bright light treatment of winter depression? The significance of hypersomnia. *Biological Psychiatry, 29*(2), 117–126. https://doi.org/10.1016/0006-3223(91)90040-s

Avery, D. H., Khan, A., Dager, S. R., Cox, G. B., & Dunner, D. L. (1990). Bright light treatment of winter depression: morning versus evening light. *Acta Psychiatrica Scandinavica, 82*(5), 335–338. https://doi.org/10.1111/j.1600-0447.1990.tb01397.x

Bond, G. R., & Drake, R. E. (2015). The critical ingredients of assertive community treatment. *World psychiatry : official journal of the World Psychiatric Association (WPA), 14*(2), 240–242. https://doi.org/10.1002/wps.20234

Ciechanowski, P., Wagner, E., Schmaling, K., Schwartz, S., Williams, B., Diehr, P., Kulzer, J., Gray, S., Collier, C., & LoGerfo, J. (2004). Community-integrated home-based depression treatment in older adults: a randomized controlled trial. *JAMA, 291*(13), 1569–1577. https://doi-org.offcampus.lib.washington.edu/10.1001/jama.291.13.1569

David L. Dunner. Interviewed by Thomas A. Ban for the ANCP, Waikoloa, Hawaii, December 13, 2001

Doug Zatzick, MD. (n.d.). Retrieved May 23, 2020, from https://academyhealth.org/about/people/doug-zatzick-md

Douglas F. Zatzick, MD. (n.d.). Retrieved May 23, 2020, from https://www.rand.org/pubs/authors/z/zatzick_douglas_f.html

Farrell, M., & Roth, B. (2013). Pharmacosynthetics: Reimagining the pharmacogenetic approach. Brain Research, 1511, 6–20. https://doi.org/10.1016/j.brainres.2012.09.043

Goldhaber-Fiebert, J., Prince, L., Xiao, L., Lv, N., Rosas, L., Venditti, E., ... Ma, J. (2020). First-Year Economic and Quality of Life Effects of the RAINBOW Intervention to Treat Comorbid Obesity and Depression. Obesity, 28(6), 1031–1039. https://doi.org/10.1002/oby.22805

John F. Neumaier, MD, PhD. (n.d.). Retrieved May 23, 2020, from https://depts.washington.edu/mnsl/john.html

Kopelovich, S., Strachan, E., Sivec, H., & Kreider, V. (2019). Stepped Care as an implementation and service delivery model for cognitive behavioral therapy for psychosis. Community Mental Health Journal, 55(5), 755–767. https://doi.org/10.1007/s10597-018-00365-6

Krupski, A., West, I., Scharf, D., Hopfenbeck, J., Andrus, G., Joesch, J., & Snowden, M. (2016, July 1). Full Access Integrating Primary Care Into Community Mental Health Centers: Impact on Utilization and Costs of Health Care. Retrieved May 24, 2020, from https://ps.psychiatryonline.org/doi/10.1176/appi.ps.201500424

Lydia Chwastiak, MD, MPH. (n.d.). Retrieved May 24, 2020, from https://aims.uw.edu/lydia-chwastiak-md-mph

Mark Snowden, MD, MPH. (n.d.). Retrieved May 24, 2020, from https://psychiatry.uw.edu/profile/mark-snowden/

Morse, G., Monroe-DeVita, M., York, M. M., Peterson, R., Miller, J., Hughes, M., Carpenter-Song, E., Akiba, C., & McHugo, G. J. (2020). Implementing illness management and recovery within assertive community treatment teams: A qualitative study. *Psychiatric rehabilitation journal, 43*(2), 121–131. https://doi.org/10.1037/prj0000387

Mueser, K. T., Meyer, P. S., Penn, D. L., Clancy, R., Clancy, D. M., & Salyers, M. P. (2006). The Illness Management and Recovery program: rationale, development, and preliminary findings. *Schizophrenia bulletin, 32 Suppl 1*(Suppl 1), S32–S43. https://doi.org/10.1093/schbul/sbl022

Neumaier Lab. (n.d.). Retrieved May 23, 2020, from https://depts.washington.edu/mnsl/

Pearls Program. (n.d.). Retrieved October 12, 2020, from https://depts.washington.edu/hprc/evidence-based-programs/pearls-program/

Publications. Sunila Nair. (n.d.). Retrieved May 23, 2020, from https://www.researchgate.net/profile/Sunila_Nair

Peter Roy-Byrne | Psychiatric Medicine Associates. (n.d.). Https://Www.Psychiatricmedicine.Com/the-Team/Md-Psychiatrist/Peter-Roy-Byrne-Md-Co-Founder-Psychiatrist. Retrieved September 26, 2020, from https://www.psychiatricmedicine.com/the-team/md-psychiatrist/peter-roy-byrne-md-co-founder-psychiatrist

Roy-Byrne, P., Stein, M. B., Russo, J., Craske, M., Katon, W., Sullivan, G., & Sherbourne, C. (2005). Medical illness and response to treatment in primary care panic disorder. *General Hospital Psychiatry, 27*(4), 237–243. https://doi.org/10.1016/j.genhosppsych.2005.03.007

Sarah Kopelovich, PhD. (n.d.-a). Retrieved May 24, 2020, from https://www.brite.uw.edu/sarahkopelovich

Sarah Kopelovich, PhD. (n.d.-b). Retrieved May 24, 2020, from http://depts.washington.edu/givemed/prof-chair/holders/sarah-kopelovich-ph-d/

Snowden, M. B., Steinman, L. E., Piering, P., Rigor, S., & Yip, A. (2015). Translating PEARLS: Lessons Learned from Providers and Participants. *Frontiers in public health, 2*, 256. https://doi-org.offcampus.lib.washington.edu/10.3389/fpubh.2014.00256

Sunila Nair, MBBS, PhD. (n.d.). Retrieved May 23, 2020, from https://psychiatry.uw.edu/profile/sunila-nair-2/

Voss, W., Kaufman, E., O'Connor, S., Comtois, K., Conner, K., & Ries, R. (2013). Preventing addiction related suicide: A pilot study. Journal of Substance Abuse Treatment, 44(5), 565–569. https://doi.org/10.1016/j.jsat.2012.10.006.

Wikipedia contributors. (2020, September 8). *David L. Dunner.* Wikipedia. https://en.wikipedia.org/wiki/David_L._Dunner